Biochemical Structure
Determination by NMR

Biochemical Structure Determination by NMR

edited by

Aksel A. Bothner-By
Department of Chemistry
Carnegie-Mellon University
Pittsburgh, Pennsylvania

Jerry D. Glickson
Comprehensive Cancer Center
University of Alabama
University Station, Alabama

Brian D. Sykes
Department of Biochemistry
and MRC Group on Protein
Structure and Function
University of Alberta
Edmonton, Alberta
Canada

MARCEL DEKKER, INC.   New York and Basel

Library of Congress Cataloging in Publication Data
Main entry under title:

Biochemical structure determination by NMR.

"Expanded versions of papers presented at the Robert Rowan III Memorial
Symposium, held at Carnegie-Mellon University in Pittsburgh, 15th September,
1979" — Pref.
Includes index.
1. Nuclear magnetic resonance — Congresses. 2. Biological chemistry —
Technique — Congresses. I. Bothner-By, Aksel A., [date]. II. Glickson,
Jerry D., III. Sykes, Brian D. IV. Robert Rowan III Memorial Symposium (1979:
Carnegie-Mellon University) V. Title: Biochemical structure determination by
N.M.R. [DNLM: 1. Biochemistry — Congresses. 2. Nuclear magnetic resonance
— Congresses. QU25 B6163 1979]
QH324.9.N8B54   574.19'285   81-22055
ISBN 0-8247-1564-0   AACR2

MARCEL DEKKER, INC.
270 Madison Avenue, New York, New York 10016

Current printing (last digit):
10 9 8 7 6 5 4 3 2 1

PRINTED IN THE UNITED STATES OF AMERICA

IN MEMORIAM

Robert Rowan III, the son of Robert Rowan, Jr. and Marian Kabler Rowan, was born July 12, 1946 in Caracas, Venezuela. His family returned to the United States in 1950, and after a brief stay at Oak Ridge National Laboratory, settled in Westfield, New Jersey in 1952. Bob attended Westfield Public School, where he was active in Cub Scouts, Boy Scouts, piano, swimming, band, Little League, chorus, football, and wrestling, and met Nancy Stiles, with whom he established a great rivalry and friendship.

In 1962, Bob and his family moved to Las Cruces, New Mexico, where he completed his studies at Las Cruces High School. He was first string center for the LCHS football team, and graduated first in his high school class.

He entered Pomona College in the fall of 1964, where he majored in chemistry, played football his freshman year, and wrestled in the heavyweight class all four years. He was all conference champion in his weight class for two years. He spent most summers while in college in New Jersey. He received an NCAA scholarship and an NSF fellowship for graduate study. In June, 1968 he graduated magna cum laude from Pomona College. In June of 1968 he also married Nancy Stiles, then a chemistry major from Mt. Holyoke College.

That fall both entered graduate school in chemistry — Bob at Harvard University and Nancy at Boston University. They lived in Cambridge for five years while they were in graduate school, and took up hiking, downhill skiing, cross country skiing and white-water canoeing. Bob became instruction chairman for white-water canoeing for the Appalachian Mt. Club. Both achieved expert canoeing ratings. Bob started his graduate career as a molecular beamist in Professor D. Herschbach's group but switched to NMR research with Professor Brian Sykes after a year.

They left Cambridge in September, 1973, after completing their degrees, and went to Bob's postdoctoral position with Aksel Bothner-By at Carnegie-Mellon University in Pittsburgh. Nancy taught at CMU. On July 29, 1974, they became the parents of Marian Stiles Rowan. After another year in Pittsburgh, Bob was appointed to an Assistant Professorship at the University of Maryland in College Park. Bob and Nancy then became homeowners in New Carrollton, Maryland. Their second child, Robert William, was born on March 31, 1977. Bob died on September 21, 1978 of cancer of the small bowel.

PREFACE

This book consists of expanded versions of papers presented at the Robert Rowan III Memorial Symposium, held at Carnegie-Mellon University in Pittsburgh, 15th September 1979. The meeting was a tribute and memorial to Robert Rowan III, whose biography appears on page iii.

Biochemical structure determination by NMR was Robert Rowan III's central interest, and his activities and collaborations affected many people, and touched many subjects. Many of his friends and colleagues participated in the symposium and presented work in areas of great current interest related to this topic. In this book have been assembled selections of those works encompassing researches on peptide and protein structure, metal-ion binding, nucleic acid structures, membrane structure and function, and whole organelles. The presentations are more complete than was possible in the short time available at the symposium and include background and perspective, such that they provide concise, instructive pictures of current frontiers.

The editors would also like to express their appreciation of the unselfish and enthusiastic response, both from the participants at the symposium and from the contributors to this volume.

We are most indebted to Ms. M. Geraci, who prepared the text files for computer-assisted photocomposition of this book, and watched over their conversion to camera-ready copy. Her dedicated work was invaluable.

Aksel A. Bothner-By
Jerry D. Glickson
Brian D. Sykes

CONTENTS

CONTRIBUTORS

IAN M. ARMITAGE, Department of Molecular Biophysics and Biochemistry, Yale University, New Haven, Connecticut

M. LOUISE BLEAM,* Department of Chemistry, University of Wisconsin, Madison, Wisconsin

ROBERT G. BRYANT, Department of Chemistry, University of Minnesota, Minneapolis, Minnesota

SUNNEY I. CHAN, Division of Chemistry and Chemical Engineering, California Institute of Technology, Pasadena, California

WILLIAM R. CROASMUN, Division of Chemistry and Chemical Engineering, California Institute of Technology, Pasadena, California

JOSEPH A. DIVERDI, Department of Chemistry, University of Pennsylvania, Philadelphia, Pennsylvania

KENNETH E. EIGENBERG,† Department of Chemistry, California Institute of Technology, Pasadena, California

FRANK R.N. GURD, Department of Chemistry, Indiana University, Bloomington, Indiana

---

*Present affiliation: Department of Chemistry, Central College, Pella, Iowa.
†Present affiliation: Research Department, Monsanto Agricultural Products Co., St. Louis, Missouri.

LANA LEE, Department of Biochemistry and MRC Group on Protein Structure and Function, University of Alberta, Edmonton, Alberta, Canada

GEORGE NEIREITER, JR., Pharmaceutical Quality Control, Mead Johnson and Company, Evansville, Indiana

STANLEY J. OPELLA, Department of Chemistry, University of Pennsylvania, Philadelphia, Pennsylvania

JAMES D. OTVOS,* Department of Molecular Biophysics and Biochemistry, Yale University, New Haven, Connecticut

DINSHAW J. PATEL, Department of Polymer Chemistry, Bell Laboratories, Murray Hill, New Jersey

M. THOMAS RECORD, JR., Department of Chemistry, University of Wisconsin, Madison, Wisconsin

DENI M. ROSE,† Department of Chemistry, University of Minnesota, Minneapolis, Minnesota

T. MICHAEL ROTHGEB,‡ School of Chemical Sciences, University of Illinois, Urbana, Illinois

KENNETH B. SEAMON, Laboratory of Bioorganic Chemistry, National Institute of Arthritis, Metabolism, and Digestive Diseases, National Institutes of Health, Bethesda, Maryland

BRIAN D. SYKES, Department of Biochemistry and MRC Group of Protein Structure and Function, University of Alberta, Edmonton, Alberta, Canada

---

*Present affiliation: Department of Chemistry, University of Wisconsin, Milwaukee, Wisconsin.

†Present affiliation: Engineering Research Center, Western Electric Co., Princeton, New Jersey.

‡Present affiliation: Ivorydale Technical Center, The Procter & Gamble Company, Cincinnati, Ohio.

Contributors

P.A. TOVO,* Department of Chemistry, University of Minnesota, Minneapolis, Minnesota

RICHARD T. WITTEBORT,† Department of Chemistry, Indiana University, Bloomington, Indiana

*Present affiliation: Honeywell Corporation, Minneapolis, Minnesota.

†Present affiliation: National Magnet Laboratory, Massachusetts Institute of Technology, Cambridge, Massachusetts.

Biochemical Structure Determination by NMR

CHAPTER 1

MOTIONS OF ALIPHATIC RESIDUES IN MYOGLOBINS

Frank R. N. Gurd, Richard J. Wittebort*
Department of Chemistry
Indiana University
Bloomington, Indiana

T. Michael Rothgeb†
School of Chemical Sciences
University of Illinois
Urbana, Illinois

George Neireiter, Jr.
Department of Pharmaceutical Quality Control
Mead Johnson and Company
Evansville, Indiana

The ability of nuclear magnetic resonance methods to observe the behavior of individual nuclei in a protein makes possible the most direct analysis of motions within the protein. Other methods that contribute to the analysis of the motional behavior of proteins include solvent exchange [1,2], fluorescence quenching and depolarization [3,4], dynamical modeling [5,6] and crystallographic analysis [7,9]. A consistent general picture emerges from all these approaches in which motions are seen to be widespread within globular proteins and even within fibrous proteins [10,11]. The particular contribution of NMR methods is to make possible the

---

* Present affiliation: National Magnet Laboratory, Massachusetts Institute of Technology, Cambridge, Massachusetts

† Present affiliation: Ivorydale Technical Center, The Proctor & Gamble Company, Cincinnati, Ohio

direct analysis of rotational motions of elements of backbone and side chains. In principle the observation can yield concurrent information at many or all points within the protein in terms of amplitudes and time scales for motion of individual structural elements. This type of information is specific and can reflect a range of time scales, and so stands in useful contrast with the types of information accumulated by the other techniques mentioned above [10,12].

Two broad types of information with respect to motions have been obtained from NMR measurements. They derive either from exchange processes in which the passage from one magnetic environment to another is observed or from nuclear relaxation processes. Probably the most useful observations of exchange processes in proteins have yielded information about flips of aromatic residues [13,14]. Much general information has come from temperature-dependent narrowing of resonances [15]. The majority of exchange processes in proteins have been observed by ^{1}H NMR, although ^{13}C NMR is also appropriate for many such purposes.

Relaxation observations of proton-decoupled ^{13}C nuclei present a particularly powerful approach for the analysis of motions of aliphatic residues in proteins. The aliphatic residues glycine, alanine, proline, valine, leucine, isoleucine and methionine are prominent in most proteins. In sperm whale myoglobin, for example, these residues constitute 69 out of the total of 153 residues in the protein. In addition the 4 methylene carbons in the side chain of lysine confer some degree of aliphatic properties on this important amino acid residue, of which there are 19 in the sperm whale myoglobin molecule. The distribution of the aliphatic residues within the protein places substantial proportions both in the interior and on the exterior of the molecule [16-18]. Indeed, virtually every residue in the protein that is not itself aliphatic makes contact with such a residue.

The nonpolar residues are not affected directly by polar constraints such as those imposed by hydrogen bonds or other electrostatic interactions, and so are free to slip past other residues [10,19,20]. Characteristically their carbon atoms are bonded to 1, 2 or 3 hydrogen atoms so that, at any but the highest magnetic fields, the [1]H-^{13}C dipolar relaxation process dominates [21]. If each carbon in a given side chain can be observed individually, it will be possible in principle to evaluate the motional behavior at each stage of the side chain in terms of the characteristics of rotational motions reorienting each [1]H-^{13}C vector. In the simplest terms these reorienting contributions are cumulative in the sense that as one considers H-C units further out a given side chain the contributions of motions affecting the more inward units are expressed in addition to those specific to the more outward units. A complete, self-consistent description of the motions of the whole residue is a potential if difficult objective.

The problem of analyzing the component elements of motion in a protein residue is illustrated in Figure 1 for the case of a lysine side chain attached to a large molecule [22,23]. For myoglobin the cylindrical symmetry appropriate for a single helical backbone can be replaced with spherical symmetry reflected in a single overall reorientation process [19,24]. The rotational motions executed by the side chain can be described in terms of rate (diffusion constant or correlation time) and amplitude of the motion about the individual C-C segments [23]. If the backbone segments of the protein are largely constrained to a relatively rigid framework, C^{α} may experience rotational motion characteristic of the overall rotational tumbling of the protein. In this simplifying case the side chain motions are accumulated in addition to the motion experienced by C^{α}. For example, C^{β} experiences the overall tumbling controlling C^{α} to which it is attached and in addition its ^{1}H-^{13}C vectors are affected by

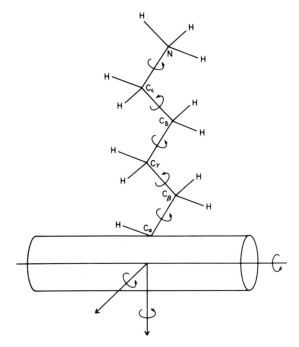

Figure 1. A lysine side chain attached to a large macromolecule of cylindrical symmetry. Taken from Wittebort and Szabo [22,23].

rotational motion about the C^α-C^β bond. For C^γCd the added effect of rotation about the C^β-C^γ bond must be taken into account.

Wallach proposed a model for the NMR relaxation process in which the side chain n-alkyl carbons are assumed to be undergoing consecutive independent and free axial diffusion-like motions about the C-C bonds [25]. This model requires adjustment because the assumption of free axial motions leads to an unrealistically large allowed conformational space. Appreciable conformational volume is excluded by collision of the side chain with itself or with the backbone. The Wallach model has recently been generalized by Wittebort and Szabo [23] to incorporate excluded volume effects by restricting the amplitude of internal rotations and independently, by London and Avitabile [26] for the case of a single internal rotation. Wittebort et al. [27] have further extended the model to allow C^α to possess a distribution of rotational correlation times to allow for the relaxation of rigid constraints in the backbone in the case of poly-L-lysine.

The present discussion will make use of the restricted diffusion treatment of Wittebort and Szabo [23] for a number of aliphatic residues in myoglobin and will attempt to show the potential scope of these applications. To set a target the poly-L-lysine case will be presented first to illustrate a reasonably complete test of the potentialities of the treatment for the n-alkyl chains. After that two aliphatic residue types will be explored, isoleucine and methionine. Isoleucine represents a branched side chain and methionine an unbranched one. Several isoleucine residues can be examined by ^{13}C NMR in myoglobin, and their behavior can therefore be taken to report on the motional processes in a substantial range of environments within the protein. Isoleucine is of special interest because the $C^{\delta 1}$ resonance can be distinguished in the natural abundance spectrum and each residue can be identified with a discrete resonance. Methionine is of special interest because it is possible to introduce substantial enrichment with respect to ^{13}C or ^{2}H in the C^ϵ position [28] so that this residue can be monitored by NMR techniques following a mild cycle of chemical treatment that does not disrupt the covalent structure of the myoglobin. The recent application of this methodology to solid state NMR experiments will also be outlined [29,30]. Both the isoleucine and methionine residues in myoglobin are largely buried within the protein matrix out of contact with solvent. It is convenient to follow their consideration by dealing with evidence for rotational motion in side chains of heme as represented by ^{2}H NMR of [^{2}H$_6$]-diacetyldeuterohemin myoglobin [31]. Lastly, a relatively mobile segment of the backbone will be examined through the replacement of the NH$_2$-terminal residue with [^{13}C-2] glycine in which C^α is enriched [32].

I. METHODOLOGY

The ^{13}C NMR spectra were obtained on two homebuilt spectrometers operating at either 15.01 MHz or 67.9 MHz. Quadrature detection was employed in the high frequency spectrometer and single phase detection in the low frequency spectrometer [27,28]. In addition a commercial spectrometer operating at 25 MHz, the Varian XL-100 was employed for certain purposes. In each case reported here the methodology will be found in the initial publication if not detailed here.

Relaxation studies were done by the inversion recovery method, i.e. by $180°$-τ-$90°$ pulse sequences. T_1 values were determined by fitting the intensities, $I(\tau)$ of each NMR line to the function $I(\tau) = A + Be$-τ/T_1 using a nonlinear least squares fitting program [27]. Proton decoupling was achieved by various procedures according to the instrument. Nuclear Overhauser enhancements, NOE, were measured at 67.9 MHz using the gated decoupling method, with a recycle time of 4.0 s, and error analysis yielded estimates of upper and lower uncertainty limits under appropriate conditions [27].

Assignment of each ^{13}C resonance was made either by comparison with model pentapeptides containing the residue in question in the central position flanked by glycine residues [33,35], by comparisons between myoglobins of appropriate animal species to obtain residue substitutions [36], by computation of chemical shifts from three-dimensional structural information [37], by adjustment of proton decoupling conditions [38], by introducing nonbinding paramagnetic species into the solvent [28], or by specific enrichment with respect to isotope [28,31,32,39].

II. LYSINE RESIDUES

The results of a recent study [27] of poly-L-lysine are interpretable in terms of a model in which the backbone carbons, C^α, are characterized by a distribution of correlation times, or diffusion constants, and the side chain carbons, C^β, C^γ, C^δ and C^ϵ, undergo independent axial motions with *restricted* amplitude. The material used in this work was polymerized to the approximate degree of $(Lys)_{129}$. The polymer tends to form both α-helical and β structures at high pH. Because of overlapping spectral components when both these structures are represented, it was found preferable to investigate the ^{13}C NMR of the poly-L-lysine at 3°C and pH 10.7, conditions that produce a primarily disordered structure according to circular dichroism criteria [27]. The ^{13}C NMR observations yielded T_1

(Figure 2) and NOE (Figure 3) measurements at 67.9 MHz, and T_1 data were also obtained at 15.1 MHz. The T_1 and NOE results are collected in Table I.

The results for C^α indicate an NOE of 1.6 ± 0.2 which is far removed from the minimum value of 1.153 that would be expected for the overall diffusional motion of a rigidly structured polypeptide backbone of 129 residues [27]. Accordingly the results were treated in terms of two para-

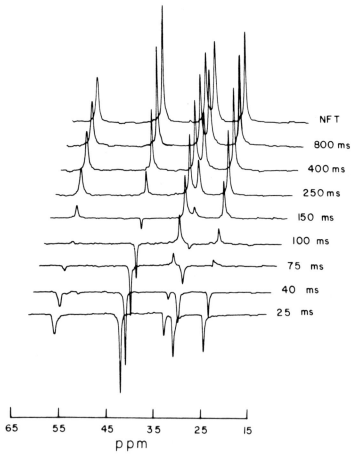

Figure 2. The 67.9 MHz inversion recovery set for (Lys)$_{129}$ obtained at 3°C and pH 10.67. The delay time between 180° pulses was 3 s. Taken from Wittebort et al. [27].

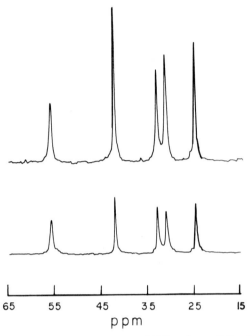

Figure 3. Spectra used for determining the NOE values of (Lys)$_{129}$ at pH 10.67 and 3°C. The spectra were obtained with continuous (upper trace) and gated (lower trace) broad band proton decoupling. The interval between 90° pulses was 4 s. Taken from Wittebort [22].

TABLE I

Measured NT$_1$ and NOE Values

| Carbon | 67.9 MHz | | 15.1 MHz |
	NT_1 (ms)	NOE[a]	NT_1 (ms)
C$^\alpha$	170 ± 8	1.6 ± 0.2	36 ± 3
C$^\beta$	202 ± 8	2.0 ± 0.2	72 ± 11
C$^\gamma$	264 ± 12	2.4 ± 0.2	108 ± 11
C$^\delta$	430 ± 20	2.3 ± 0.2	208 ± 23
C$^\epsilon$	734 ± 50	2.7 ± 0.2	484 ± 69

[a] NOE is defined as $(1 + \psi)$. Taken from Wittebort et al. [27].

meters, D_L and D_U, which are respectively the lower and upper limits of a diffusional constant distribution. It was found that the two observed values for T_1 measured at different frequencies (Table I) uniquely specified D_L and D_U. Furthermore, the parameter values $D_L = 2.5 \times 10^6$ s^{-1} and $D_U = 5.0 \times 10^8$ s^{-1} lead to a predicted NOE value at 67.9 MHz of 1.6 in agreement with that observed (Table I).

The relaxation data for the lysyl side chain C^β, C^γ, C^δ, and C^ϵ, were analyzed in terms of the established backbone motional behavior and for two models of consecutive internal reorientation. It was easily shown [27] that the results are not fit consistently at the two spectrometer frequencies if it is assumed that each of the internal motions is an independent, axial, diffusion process. In this model, for example, a ^{13}C-^1H vector of C, viewed from C^δ is viewed as simply undergoing rotational diffusion about the C^δ-C^ϵ bond axis with diffusion constant D_ϵ. Similarly, the C^δ is rotationally diffusing about the C^γ-C^δ bond axis with diffusion constant D_δ when viewed from C^γ, and so on. Since in this model a rotation about, say, the C^β-C^γ bond not only reorients a C^γ-H vector but also the C^δ-H and C^ϵ-H vectors, the diffusion constants can be expected to increase monotonically towards the end of the side chain, i.e. $D_\beta < D_\gamma < D_\delta < D_\epsilon$. This inadequate model was readily fit from T_1 values for C^β, C^γ, C^δ and C^ϵ observed at only a single spectrometer frequency, but the computations for the two frequencies studied could not be reconciled [27]. It was found, for example, that the diffusion constants, with the exception of D_ϵ were a factor of 2 greater when determined at 15.1 MHz. The NOE values in Table I likewise failed to agree with those computed from the T_1 data at 67.9 MHz according to the unrestricted internal rotational model.

A successful fit of the T_1 and NOE data of Table I was obtained by allowing for excluded volume effects resulting from the inability of the side chain to crossover on itself or occupy the same volume as the peptide backbone. This was done by restricting the amplitudes of the internal rotations to occur within a specified angular region [23,27]. This restriction has the effect of decreasing the T_1 value computed at lower frequencies such as 15.1 MHz for a given diffusion constant. In this case for each D_i, a corresponding angular parameter γ_i is determined such that a unique pair of D_i and γ_i values will simultaneously reproduce both high and low frequency T_1 data for the corresponding carbon atom. The results in Table II show that the requirements for good fit at both spectrometer frequencies are met by this procedure. In addition, the theoretical NOE values agree with those determined experimentally. In the present instance restriction of diffusion about the C^δ-C^ϵ bond was not introduced. The fit could likely be improved by introducing such a restriction; in molecular

TABLE II

Calculated Amplitudes, Diffusion Constants and NOE and T_1 Values from the Restricted Diffusion Model[a]

Carbon	$\pm \gamma_i$ (degrees)	Best Fit $D_i (10^9 s^{-1})$	67.9 MHz NOE Calculated (experiment)	67.9 MHz T_1 (MS) Calculated (experiment)	15.1 MHz T_1 (MS) Calculated (experiment)
C^β	$\pm 60°$	1.0	2.13 (2.0±0.2)	205 (202± 8)	69 (72±11)
C^γ	$\pm 50°$	1.5	2.40 (2.4±0.2)	254 (264± 12)	117 (108± 11)
C^δ	$\pm 120°$	3.3	2.55 (2.3±0.2)	409 (430± 20)	224 (208± 23)
C^ϵ	–	3.3	2.86 (2.7± 0.2)	680 (734± 50)	574 (484± 70)

[a] Taken from Wittebort et al. [27].

terms some such allowance for the effect of the bulky hydrated ammonium group is reasonable.

The values for the calculated amplitudes of internal rotation shown in Table II are qualitatively reasonable in terms of the postulated excluded volume effects. Crossovers within the side chain, exclusion from the backbone space and collision with other residue segments presumably shape the observed results on the disordered poly-L-lysine [22,23]. The results for 15.1 MHz in Table I may be compared for the C^α and C^ϵ, respectively, with those for the pentapeptide containing the lysine residue flanked on both sides by two glycine residues, at 28°: 180, 242, 432, 672 and 960 ms [35]. In the case of the small peptide the effective overall rotational diffusion time should be significantly shorter. Similarly, the pentapeptide presents fewer restrictions from neighboring segments on the amplitude of angular reorientations in the lysine side chain. Conversely, the T_1 of 484 ms measured for C^ϵ of polylysine is larger than the value of 278 ms measured at the same frequency by Glushko et al. for lysine C^ϵ resonances in ribonuclease [40,41]. In denatured carboxymethyl myoglobin a value of 182 ms for the T_1 has been observed at the same frequency, and shorter values in the range 108-120 ms have been observed for native myoglobins [42]. The results indicate a more restricted mobility of the lysine residues in the protein.

The results with polylysine show that the simple model adapted by Wittebort et al. [27] from the general treatment of Wittebort and Szabo [23] describes adequately the motional behavior of the 4-carbon side chain anchored to a disordered, flexible backbone. The model suggests, reasonably, a substantial limitation on the amplitude of rotation around the C^α-C^β and C^β-C^γ bonds with a lesser restriction around the C^γ-C^δ bond, and could probably be somewhat better fit if some restriction were introduced for the C^δ-C^ϵ bond. Although the packing density in proteins varies somewhat in different regions [43] the general density is normal for an organic material [47,44]. It is to be expected, therefore, that in a protein aliphatic chain such as that of lysine will be relatively more hindered by the neighboring side chains, especially the branched side chains, than in polylysine itself. On the other hand, x-ray structural evidence often shows the outer segments of lysine chains protruding from the neighboring surface region of a protein [10,16,18,45]. The polylysine case, therefore, serves to illustrate the unbranched chain case in a structure that is probably somewhat less restricted especially close to the backbone than we should expect in a protein.

Note that in Table II the rotational diffusion constants for all stages imply correlation times of the order of 0.1 to 1 ns. The side chain diffusion constants are greater than D_U, the upper limit of the range applying to C^α, as required for them to be distinguished from the overall diffusive motion. As can be pictured with the aid of Figure 1, the displacements of side chain atoms, C^γ, C^δ, C^ϵ, N^ζ relative to C^α can be large in tracing out the motions described above. Some of the indicated rotational activity can be accommodated by cranking motions in which certain axes are relatively free and others are temporarily nearly locked, thus confining the side chain to a smaller overall motional space. Since the individual lysine residues in polylysine exist in substantially equivalent environments all corresponding carbon atoms will experience similar magnetic environments over a short period of time and will represent in the aggregate a single behavior with respect to the NMR spectrum. Although the same may hold true for practical purposes for the outermost carbons of many lysine residues in proteins, it is unlikely to apply among the inner carbons of the side chain.

III. ISOLEUCINE RESIDUES

The isoleucine residue has a branched aliphatic side chain in which the C^β bears one branch consisting of $C^{\gamma 1}$ and $C^{\delta 1}$ and another consisting of $C^{\gamma 2}$. Almost all isoleucine residues in myoglobins occur in α-helical regions of the polypeptide sequence. The helical backbone arrangement and the β-fork structure of the side chain produce an extreme example of constraint of rotational motion about the C^α-C^β bond axis, to a total amplitude of less than 30°. Unless this constraint can be partially relieved by flexing of the helical backbone or significant bond distortion, the amplitude of rotational motions about the C^α-C^β bond will be so limited by collision of $C^{\gamma 1}$ and $C^{\gamma 2}$ with elements of the backbone that this motional mode will not contribute to the dipolar NMR relaxation process which requires each single axial diffusion process to have a total amplitude of 40° ($\pm$ 20°) or more [38]. In this way the ^{13}C-^1H dipolar vector of C^β will be locked in a fixed relationship with that of C^α for practical purposes. While the methyl groups spinning about the C^β-$C^{\gamma 2}$ and $C^{\gamma 1}$-$C^{\delta 1}$ axes may be almost totally unhindered, one element of shape change is left to the isoleucine side chain, namely, that of reorientation about the C^β-$C^{\gamma 1}$ bond axis. Here again certain limits are placed on rotation about the C^β-$C^{\gamma 1}$ bond; if the side chain is in a *trans*, $\chi_{2,1} = 180°$, configuration, rotation about the C^β-$C^{\gamma 1}$ bond is limited to an extent of 80° in either direction by collisions of the $C^{\delta 1}$ methyl group with the backbone. Within these constraints internal diffusive rotations are allowed about the C^β-$C^{\gamma 1}$ and $C^{\gamma 1}$-$C^{\delta 1}$ bonds with correlation times τ_{g1} and τ_{g2}, respectively. For physical reasons it is required that $\tau_{g1} < \tau_{g2}$ [38]. We shall refer to the restriction on rotation about the C^β-$C^{\gamma 1}$ bond as imposing limits to $\pm$ γ_0, and we expect $\gamma_0 \lesssim$ 80°. In the limit of $\gamma_0 \lesssim$ 20° this model is independent of τ_{g1} and is equivalent to a single degree of internal reorientation for the ^{13}C-^1H vectors in the $C^{\delta 1}$ methyl group, a situation comparable to that of the $C^{\gamma 2}$ methyl group. On the other hand if γ_0 could reach 180°, the model would be similar to that of two degrees of unrestricted and uncorrelated internal reorientation. In practice we expect the limit of $\gamma_0 \lesssim$ 80° to hold and to be potentially reduced in practice by diffusional collision of $C^{\delta 1}$ with elements of the protein structure other than its own immediate backbone elements.

Eight single carbon resonances are observed for sperm whale cyanoferrimyoglobin in the spectral region from 9 to 15 ppm and can be assigned to $C^{\delta 1}$ of 8 of the 9 isoleucine residues in sperm whale myoglobin [46]. This class assignment is made on the basis of ^{13}C NMR of peptide models [33] and is supported by comparative studies of myoglobins containing various isoleucine substitutions as referred to below. The pertinent region of the spectrum is illustrated in Figure 4 by convolution difference spectra representing, respectively, continuous and gated proton decoupling [38]. The lower spectrum shows each resonance to represent an equal number of ^{13}C nuclei, and reference to the corresponding intensity for the full α-carbon envelope proves this number to be 1 carbon atom per resonance in the region of 9 to 15 ppm. The upper spectrum in Figure 4 indicates the particular degrees of NOE.

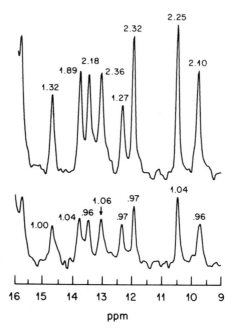

Figure 4. Convolution difference spectra of the eight resonances in the 9 to 15 ppm region. The differences were taken between a spectrum with 5-Hz digital broadening and the same spectrum with 50-Hz broadening, its vertical scale decreased by a factor of 0.7. The upper trace is from the continuous proton decoupled spectrum and the lower trace from the gated decoupled spectrum. The numbers indicate the integrated intensity of each resonance normalized such that the eight resonances in the lower trace have an integral of 8.0. Taken from Wittebort et al. [38].

The range of chemical shifts shown in Figure 4 establishes that the magnetic environments of the isoleucine $C^{\delta 1}$ are distinct. The methods used to assign the resonances to particular residues are summarized in Table III [T.M. Rothgeb, R.J. Wittebort, A. Szabo and F.R.N. Gurd, in preparation]. With one exception, to be discussed below, the computed pseudocontact contributions [10,28] to the ^{13}C chemical shift values fitted well with the temperature dependence of the observed chemical shifts, largely because in all such cases the relationship of the isoleucine residue to the paramagnetic heme dominated the various contributions to the shift. Single frequency proton decoupling experiments were confirmatory. Temperature dependence of the chemical shifts was used to establish that the resonance of residue 107 was sufficiently influenced by paramagnetic

TABLE III

Basis of Assignments of Isoleucine $C^{\delta 1}$ Resonances

Chemical shift ppm	Residue assignment	Computed shifts, decoupling frequencies, temperature dependence	Preferential paramagnetic broadening	Comparisons between species
14.16	28			X
13.17	30	X	X	
12.85	112	X	X	
12.51	111			X
11.75	107[a]	X		
11.40	142			X
9.80	101		X	
9.20	75	X		

[a] Relaxation process not dominated by dipolar coupling mechanism (see text and Table IV).

relaxation effects that it could not be used to evaluate motional behavior of the resonance (Table III). Likewise, the $C^{\delta 1}$ resonance for residue 99, not visible in Figure 2, was shown to be excessively influenced by paramagnetic effects to provide motional information. These $C^{\delta 1}$ nuclei are located 6.7 angstroms and 6.3 angstroms, respectively, from the iron atom of the heme [18], and so the relaxation behavior could readily be influenced by the paramagnetic heme.

The assignments of residues 30, 112 and 101 were made on the basis of preferential paramagnetic broadening of the resonances by the introduction of an unbound free radical in the same way as had been done previously to distinguish C^ϵ of the two methionine residues in sperm whale myoglobin [28]. In these experiments the degree of line broadening could be correlated with the degree of exposure of the $C^{\delta 1}$ methyl groups to the aqueous solvent [28]. The recognition of residues 28, 111 and 142 was made by comparison of the sperm whale myoglobin spectrum with those of the myoglobins of man [47], common porpoise [48] and dwarf sperm whale [49]. In the case of residue 142 the resonance position of $C^{\delta 1}$ implies that the relationship with the nearby ring of Phe-138 is somewhat changed relative to the structure in the crystalline state. Although the motion of these side chains relative to each other cannot be specified, such motions do most certainly exist [10].

Having completed the isoleucine $C^{\delta 1}$ resonance assignments it is possible to combine them with the intepretation of $C^{\delta 1}$ T_1 and NOE values to gain information concerning the individual side chain environments [38]. Values for NT_1, where N is the number of directly bonded hydrogens, here equal to 3, and NOE values for the pertinent resonances have been reported for 30°C [38] and are summarized in Table IV. Within the framework of the model for motions of the isoleucine residue outlined above, four phenomenological constants are required to be uniquely determined by the experimental measurements: τ_R, the rotational correlation time for overall tumbling, τ_{g1} and τ_{g2}, the rotational correlation times for rotation about C^β-$C^{\gamma 1}$ and $C^{\gamma}1$-$C^{\delta 1}$, respectively, and γ_0, the angular limits within which rotation about C^β-$C^{\gamma}1$ is restricted. The value for τ_R is supplied by observations on the relaxation of the α-carbon envelope, for which T_1 is 400 ms under these conditions, which yields τ_R of 16 ns, in agreement with other measurements [19,50,51]. The sensitivity of the calculations to the various parameters is evident from Figure 5.

Values of γ_0 for each residue in Table IV were obtained along with values of τ_{g2} in the range 1 to 6 ps as unique sets of values that reproduced within 5% the experimental data in all cases. The results for residues 28 and 30 are consistent with rapid rotation only of the $C^{\delta 1}$ methyl group.

TABLE IV

Motional Parameters of Isoleucine Side Chains[a]

Residue assignment	Observed $NT_1(s)$	NOE	Theoretical γ_0
28	3.05	1.32	< 20°
30	1.95	1.82	< 20°
112	2.46	2.27	40°
111	2.34	2.23	40°
107	2.18	1.31	—
142	2.13	2.39	40°
101	2.06	2.16	30°
75	2.13	2.19	30°

[a] Measurements were made at 32°C [38]. NOE is defined as $(1 + \psi)$.

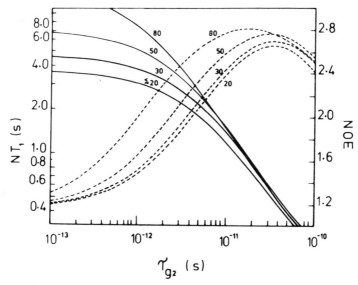

Figure 5. Explicit calculations for isoleucine motional model described in the text. The correlation time for rotation about C^{β}-$C^{\gamma 2}$, τ_{g1}, has been taken as $3\tau_{g2}$ and the rotational correlation time, τ_R, is 16 ns. The numbers on the curves refer to values of γ_0

Any additional side chain motions, if present, are such that they do not influence the $C^{\delta 1}$ relaxation behavior. The experimental values for the remaining 5 residues are consistent with two degrees of internal rotation with substantial amplitudes for rotation about C^{β}-$C^{\gamma 1}$. The amplitudes for this rotation are such that the diffusive displacement of the $C^{\delta 1}$ methyl group amounts to approximately 2 angstroms at the limits relative to the rest of the residue in the cases where γ_0 equals 40°. Separate results obtained at 52°C show with equal consistency that γ_0 now ranges between 20° (residue 30) and 50° (residues 28, 101 and 75), indicating increased diffusive mobility within the protein at the higher temperature (T.M. Rothgeb, R.J. Wittebort, A. Szabo and F.R.N. Gurd, in preparation). These results will be discussed further below. It is important to note at this point that the isoleucine residues listed in Table IV occur in a variety of environments within the myoglobin molecule.

Although it has been assumed that $\tau_{g1} = 3\tau_{g2}$ for the purpose of the calculations, there is experimental evidence for the appropriate T_1 values for resonances in the part of the ^{13}C spectrum of myoglobin to fit those to be computed for $C^{\gamma 1}$ of each isoleucine residue considered. In this computation the $C^{\gamma 1}$ is assumed to undergo rotational reorientation of the sort attributed here on the basis of the positively identified $C^{\delta 1}$ resonances [38]. In the case of the simple pentapeptide, Gly-Gly-Ile-Gly-Gly, the NT_1 value at 15.1 MHz for $C^{\delta 1}$ is 4 to 5 times longer than for $C^{\gamma 1}$ [33].

IV. METHIONINE RESIDUES

The two methionine residues, 55 and 131, carry nonpolar unbranched side chains that probe, like the isoleucine residues, the internal environments of the myoglobin. The restrictions on rotational motions within the methionine side chains are inherently much less strict than those on the isoleucine, and resemble the more simple excluded volume effects illustrated for the lysine side chain. Without full observation of all carbon resonances in the side chain, as was possible with the polylysine case, it is not possible to make a detailed analysis of the motional behavior of the methionine residues. Nevertheless, it has been possible by chemical means to enrich the C^{ϵ} methyl group with respect to ^{13}C so that it is readily examined in an otherwise crowded region of the spectrum. The results show that the relaxation behavior for both methionine C^{ϵ} nuclei reflects rotational reorientation to a significant degree about several bonds in each side chain. So far as they go these results are completely consistent with those for the isoleucine residues. In particular, the mobile isoleucine 112 side chain is in contact in the crystallographic structure with methionine 131. It is eminently reasonable that if one flexible side chain undergoes substantial diffusive motions the same will be true for a flexible neighboring side chain with which it makes direct contact in the time average structure.

The enrichment procedure [28] employed involves the opening up of the myoglobin under denaturing conditions, allowing access of $^{13}CH_3I$ to the methionine S^{δ} atoms. Under suitable conditions of reagent concentration and pH, the methionine is converted in situ to the S-methyl methionine form as the sulfonium salt bearing two substantially equivalent methyl groups, one of which is enriched to the desired degree in ^{13}C. The acid conditions make it possible to avoid methylation of other reactive nucleophiles. The process can be reversed subsequently by exposure of the still intact protein to sulfhydryl compounds such as dithiothreitol or dithioerythritol which remove nearly randomly one or the other methyl group from each S-methyl methionine residue, thereby restoring the original methionine residues now enriched to the extent of 50% of that of the $^{13}CH_3I$ that was employed in the original methylation. The protein preparation is indistinguishable otherwise from the original material [28] and indeed has been crystallized routinely [29,30].

The enriched resonances were readily observed, separated by approximately 1 ppm. The principal evidence on which the two resonances were assigned was obtained by differential paramagnetic broadening by an unbound free radical [28]. This procedure was later adapted to the isoleucine study described above. In connection with the methionine study the appropriate controls by EPR measurements and with a fixed NH_2-terminal adduct of the free radical were performed. Both the free radicals 2,2,6,6-tetramethylpiperidinooxy and its 4-hydroxy analogue produced identical results showing the slightly exposed residue 55 to be far more subject to broadening than the deeply buried residue 131.

Measurements of T_1 were made at 27-30°C at three spectrometer field strengths: 15.1, 25.2 and 67.9 MHz. It was easy to show that a simple model in which only the C^ϵ methyl group rotation was taken into account along with overall tumbling did not fit the results at all spectrometer frequencies [28]. Clearly, one or more possible rotational reorientation modes about the C^α-C^β, C^β-C^γ or C^γ-S^δ bonds was also involved with significant amplitude.

Note that the multiple potential modes of reorientation in the methionine residue stand in contrast to the limited motion of the isoleucine residue. Nevertheless, it is possible to correlate further information concerning the temperature dependence of the motion of the contiguous residues 112 (G13) and 131 (H7) forming members of the nearly parallel G and H helices, respectively. Measurements to be reported separately (T.M. Rothgeb, R. J. Wittebort, A. Szabo and F. R. N. Gurd, in preparation) on the isoleucine $C^{\delta 1}$ resonances at 52°C show that the amplitude of the half-angle γ_0 for residue 112 does not increase relative to that at 32°C (Table IV). The dominant motion involved occurs freely even at the lower temperature and the activation energy required for motion of a greater amplitude is inaccessible even at 52°C. Similarly, T_2 observations on the C^ϵ resonances of methionine residue 131 indicate an activation energy of only 2.6 ± 0.1 kcal/mol for the resonance. In both instances the motional processes accessible to the two contiguous residues involve low activation energies, exceeding the minimum for unhindered rotation about a single bond [52], thus implying relatively free diffusive motions occurring within angular displacements of ± 60°. Similar behavior is observed for methionine 55 as for 131. Isoleucine residues 30, 111 and 142 share with residue 112 the tendency to diffuse within motional limits that change little with temperature, whereas residues 28, 75 and 101 experience distinct increases in the diffusion limits for γ_0 as the temperature is raised from 32°C to 52°C.

Measurements of NT_1 for C^ϵ in the pentapeptide Gly-Gly-Met-Gly-Gly at 15.1 MHz [35] show a value somewhat exceeding that for $C^{\delta 1}$ in the corresponding isoleucine peptide [33]. The relative values are reasonable in terms of the lesser rotational restrictions inherent in the methionine residues.

The feasibility of obtaining C^ϵ methyl enrichment of methionine residues in myoglobin preparations capable of forming normal crystals opens the way for a comparison of the motional properties of these residues in the crystalline and dissolved states [29,30]. The discovery that the paramagnetic forms of myoglobin in the crystalline state respond to the primary magnetic field of the NMR spectrometer opens the way for a thorough, systematic study of the oriented crystals by the procedures of solid state NMR [30]. To illustrate the spectra obtainable from crystals of myoglobin in which the methionine methyl groups are enriched with -C^2H_3, the following results are shown in Figure 6 [30]. The clarity of detail

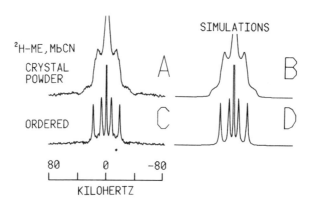

Figure 6. Deuterium quadrupole-echo Fourier transform NMR spectra at 55.3 MHz and 22 ± 1°C of ^{2}H-methyl methionine labelled sperm whale cyanoferrimyoglobin microcrystals. A, Solid powder sample hydrated with 90% saturated $(NH_4)_2SO_4$, 233644 scans, 65 ms recycle time, $\tau_1 = \tau_2 = 65 \mu s$, 7 μs 90° pulse widths, 167 kHz spectral width, 4K real data points, linebroadening = 400 Hz. B, Spectral simulation of the result of A using $\Delta\nu_Q = 33.0$ kHz, $\psi = 0.15$, and $2\delta = 2.8$ kHz. C, Magnetically ordered cyanoferrimyoglobin suspended in ~ 90% saturated $(NH_4)_2SO_4$, pH = 6.4. 940703 scans, 61 ms recycle time, $\tau_1 = \tau_2 = 61 \mu s$, μs 90° pulse widths, 167 kHz spectral width, 4K real data points, 400 Hz linebroadening. D, Simulation of the spectrum shown in C using $\Theta_1 = 32.1$°, $\Theta_2 = 63.7$° (or 46.7°), $2\delta = 2.4$ kHz. Taken from Rothgeb and Oldfield [30].

in this figure is striking and illustrates the low background obtainable with
^{2}H-enrichment.

V. HEME PROSTHETIC GROUP

In connection with the analysis of motions of aliphatic residues in myoglobins it is useful to examine the motional characteristics of certain side
chains of the heme prosthetic group. The heme provides a reference
within the protein structure. When 4-amino-1-naphtholsulfonate is substituted for it in the protein, it is possible to determine the overall rotational
diffusion constant by studies of fluorescence behavior [53,54]. The value
obtained is in general agreement with the expectation from hydrodynamic
theory and with the estimates from the relaxation behavior of the α-
carbons [19,38,50].

Motions of the heme side chains can be probed by NMR relaxation
techniques if a quadrupolar nucleus such as ^{2}H is introduced to diminish
the sensitivity to the paramagnetism of the heme. Oster et al. [31] prepared sperm whale myoglobin substituted with 2,4-diacetyldeuterohemin
deuterated in the methyl groups of the acetyl moieties. The acetyl groups
project into the internal region of the molecule occupied in the natural
heme form by vinyl groups. The study bore out the expected relative
insensitivity of the ^{2}H resonances to paramagnetic line broadening. The
Varian HR 220 spectrometer was operated at 33.77 MHz in the pulsed
Fourier transform mode at 15-17°C in most cases. The experiments were
conducted in H_2O without enrichment with respect to ^{2}H other than in the
two methyl groups of the acetyl moieties. Taking the heme nucleus as a
reference, the motions experienced by the methyl groups are about the
axes of the bond connecting it to the carbonyl carbon and of the bond
connecting the carbonyl carbon to the heme nucleus. There is some
analogy in this case, therefore, with the principal motions of the isoleucine
side chain. Four states of the heme coordination were explored, the ferro
forms CO and O_2 and the ferri forms CN^- and H_2O (Figures 7 and 8). They
appeared to be comparably stable to the derivatives of the natural heme
form.

The characteristics of ^{2}H relaxation are such that the linewidth of a
resonance representing a $-C^2H_3$ group limited to the overall tumbling
reorientation of the protein would be approximately 1000 Hz [31]. In
practice linewidths of 20 to 30 Hz were observed. Internal rotation
accounts for much of the 40-fold narrowing observed. From T_{-1} measurements an effective correlation time for rotation about the two axes of the

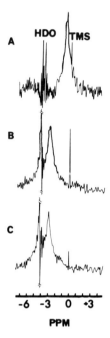

Figure 7. ^{2}H NMR spectra measured by pulsed Fourier transform spectroscopy at 33.77 MHz at 15-17°C. The protein is myoglobin prepared from sperm whale apomyoglobin and D_6-2, 4-diacetyldeuterohemin in which the methyl groups of the acetyl groups bear the deuterium atoms. A, cyanoferrimyoglobin, 5 to 6 mM, with 10-fold excess of KCN in phosphate buffer, ionic strength 0.1 M, pH 6.7. B, carbonmonoxymyoglobin, 5 to 6 mM, 0.1 M Tris-HCl buffer, pH 8.6. C, oxymyo-globin, 5 to 6 mM, 0.1 M Tris-HCl buffer, pH 8.6. External D_{12}-Me_4Si was used as a reference, and its separately recorded spectrum is overlaid by computer in each case, with chemical shifts expressed in ppm. Spectra are derived from 32768 accumulations with a recycle time of 0.211 s. Taken from Oster et al. [31].

acetyl groups would be of the order of 50 ps for each of the heme coordina-tion states. The observed values of T_1 appear to be at least an order of magnitude too large to be determined solely by the methyl group rotation [31].

Temperature dependence of the linewidths was observed to be com-parable with that already discussed for the methionine methyl groups. The variations in internal freedom within the protein molecule probably allow progressively greater freedom for the rotational reorientation of the acetyl side chains in the 2,4-diacetyldeuterohemin derivative. In explaining the

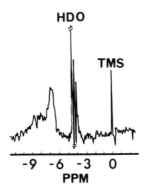

Figure 8. Spectrum corresponding to Figure 7, at 17°C. The aquoferrimyoglobin prepared from D_6-2, 4-diacetyldeuterohemin and sperm whale apomyoglobin was 6 mM, pH 6.5, in 0.1 M phosphate buffer. Other conditions are the same as in Figure 7. Taken from Oster et al. [31].

temperature dependence of the spin state equilibrium of hemoproteins, Otsuka [55] proposed a cooperative loosening of van der Waals contacts between the porphyrin and the protein moieties. In the present case the two methyl resonances in the aquoferriprotein derivative are distinct (Figure 8) rather than overlaid (Figure 7) as is otherwise the rule in this study, and one is relatively broadened. This may represent a differential restraint on rotation if paramagnetic or other effects are not responsible. Restriction of heme methyl group rotation has been invoked by Morishima and Iizuka [56]. The sensitivity of the -C^2H_3 resonances to subtle structural effects are illustrated by differences in the (overlaid) chemical shifts in passing between the oxymyoglobin, CO-myoglobin, and cyanoferrimyoglobin forms [31]. Indeed distinct effects of added phosphate and of cyclopropane, each known to affect the function or structure in the neighborhood of the heme [57-59], were clearly evident in this work. The various heme derivative forms were also found to differ measurably in their C^ϵ methionine resonance positions in the study discussed above [28].

VI. MOTIONS OF AMINO-TERMINAL BACKBONE

Examination of the results of measurement of the relaxation of ^{13}C-enriched C^α in the amino-terminal residue of myoglobin is pertinent for two reasons. First, it can be shown that the terminal glycine residue in

[Gly][1] myoglobin experiences internal reorientation in addition to the overall molecular tumbling. Second, the semisynthetic procedure for the introduction of the complete amino acid residue bearing the isotopic enrichment represents the application of one of a variety of semisynthetic approaches that can, in principle, open the way to numerous such manipulations of isotope content or sequence.

The procedure is called semisynthetic because the natural intact protein is used as the starting material for a series of manipulations that result in the removal of the amino-terminal residue followed by recoupling of a new amino acid to replace it. Differential reactivity of α- and ϵ-amino groups was exploited [58] to prepare in good yield [59,60] a derivative of sperm whale myoglobin in which all 19 lysine ϵ-amino groups were converted to the acetimidyl form by reaction with methylacetimidate without blocking the α-amino group of the terminal valine residue. This step serves to direct coupling of the Edman reagent, 3-sulfophenyl isothiocyanate, exclusively to the α-amino group. Anhydrous trichloracetic acid is used to effect cleavage to free the α-amino of the second residue, leucine. During the anhydrous acid step the heme must be absent; it is reintroduced immediately afterwards [60,61]. Following this step, the des-Val[1]-acetimidomyoglobin is coupled with an amino-protected, activated amino acid such as the N-hydroxysuccinimide ester of methylsulfonyl-ethyloxy-carbonyl-protected L-valine. The amino-protecting groups are then removed in a single step to yield a molecule identical with the starting material with only a small amount of readily distinguishable contaminating byproduct [39,60]. The final coupling process can be varied; thus far the [Gly][1], [Lys][1], and [Glu][1] myoglobins have been characterized [39].

Separate preparations of [2-^{13}C, Gly][1] myoglobin have been obtained [32]. A representative ^{13}C-NMR spectrum is shown in Figure 9. The prominent resonance at 43.4 ppm represents the enriched C^{α} of the amino-terminal glycine residue introduced by the semisynthetic sequence of reactions. From the pH dependence of the chemical shift a pK of approximately 7.6 is computed for the α-amino group. As illustrated in Figure 10, the relaxation behavior is strongly pH dependent.

In the acid limit of full protonation of the α-amino group, below pH 6.5, the relaxation behavior could be fit with T_1 measurements at 67.9 MHz and 25.2 MHz by a single motional model. The T_1 values were too long, and the linewidths too narrow to be fit by a rigid rotational reorientation model according to the overall tumbling alone, such as serves for the envelope of the C^{α} resonances as a whole [19,38,50]. Ascribing a single internal reorientation about the C^{α}-C° axis of the terminal glycine residue

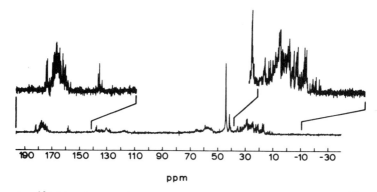

Figure 9. ^{13}C Fourier transform proton coupled NMR spectrum of [2-^{13}C,Gly^1] cyanoferrimyoglobin at pH 7.3, 30°C. The ppm scale is referenced to external Me$_4$Si. The spectrum resulted from 8192 accumulations at a recycle time of 4 s. The ^{1}H decoupler was centered at 2.5 ppm downfield of Me$_4$Si and 1000 Hz noise modulation bandwidth applied. The resonance of C$^\alpha_1$ dominates the spectrum at 43.4 ppm. The expanded regions downfield and upfield of the C$^\alpha_1$ resonance are provided to show more clearly the resonances due to C° at 170 to 185 ppm, C$^\zeta$ of arginines and tyrosines at about 158 ppm, and the C$^{\delta\gamma}$ of isoleucines at 10 to 15 ppm (see Figure 4). These last resonances were identical in chemical shift, within digital resolution, between the semisynthetic and virgin cyanoferrimyoglobin [38]. Taken from Neireiter [32].

was likewise insufficient. A successful model was developed by Lipari and Szabo [62] whereby, rather than confining the internal motion to diffusional rotation about one bond, the ^{13}C-^{1}H vector is viewed as wandering inside a cone of a given semiangle [32]. The choice of this model for investigation derives from the lack of rigidity of the backbone elements of both the first and second residues in the crystal structures of the sperm whale and harbor seal myoglobins [63], which represent protein species in which these residues are Val-Leu- and Gly-Leu-, respectively [46,64]. The model reflects to some degree a limitation on the internal reorientation contributed by the backbone segment comprising the second residue. The treatment according to this model has not necessarily reached its final form, but it is consistent at the two spectrometer frequencies and describes an effective correlation time for reorientation around the C$^\alpha$-C° axis of the terminal glycine residue of approximately 25 ps. This value is comparable to that computed for a simple pentapeptide of sequence identical with that of the terminal sequence of the semisynthetic protein [32]. This fact implies that the internal motions of the NH$_2$-terminus of the protein are

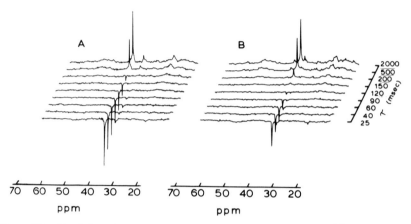

Figure 10.   Partially relaxed Fourier transform proton decoupled ^{13}C NMR spectra of [2-^{13}C,Gly^1] aquoferrimyoglobin at pH 9.2 (A) and pH 6.3 (B). The delay times, τ, in the inversion-recovery technique are shown next to each spectrum, in each case with 300 accumulations with a recycle time of 2 s. Note that at $\tau = 200$ ms the C$^\alpha{}_1$ resonance is inverted at pH 9.2 and upright at pH 6.3, reflecting a longer T_1 indicating greater motional freedom of the deprotonated residue. Taken from Neireiter [32].

not severely restricted by the remainder of the protein beyond the first few residues [32]. Clearly, the motion of C$^\alpha$ of the terminal residue is uncharacteristic of the typical α-carbons in the protein [19,32,38,50]. The motional behavior at higher pH, where the uncharged α-amino form comes to dominate, is more complex and no model has yet been developed for it. It is clear, however, that at the higher pH motional constraints on the amino-terminal residue are further relaxed.

VII. DISCUSSION

The foregoing set of probes of internal motion of aliphatic and related residues in myoglobins provide some view of the widespread nature of motions within these proteins. The molecule is close-packed with the normal overall packing density within the usual range of 0.70 - 0.75 [17,43,44]. In general therefore, diffusion of one motional element such as the twisting of a side chain or backbone segment implies some complementary motions of neighboring structures within the molecule. The aliphatic residues are particularly interesting because their side chains are devoid of the adherence provided by polar interactions and hence readily slip by each other to allow displacements that can encompass a number of side chains together.

Myoglobins contain two main nonpolar pools of side chains on either side of the heme extending below it away from the border that carries the heme propionic acid residues. These pools communicate below the lower heme border or by relative displacements of the heme itself. At various points within the time-average structure probed by X-ray diffraction evidence can be found for small cavities, possibly connecting, whose existence is compatible with the evidence for the motility of the protein matrix if not required by it [12,17,43,44]. The time-average existence of small cavities is probably directly related to the passage of O_2 through the protein matrix from the outside to reach the heme iron site where it is bound and from which it escapes again into the surroundings. Relatively small displacements are required to bring these cavities into continuous contact as channels for the penetration processes. Nevertheless, to accommodate the O_2 molecule displacements of 2 to 3 angstroms are required and will involve substantial transient deviations from the time average structure. To the extent that the motions of contiguous structural elements are concerted, it is useful to consider the nonpolar pool regions as "domains" [10,13,14,65]. An important indication of motility within such a domain has been the observation of flips of aromatic side chains as a function of temperature [10,13,14].

In the nonpolar pool or pocket on the O_2-binding side of the heme in myoglobin are found the following residues whose motions have been discussed: Ile-28, Ile-30, Met-55, Ile-101, Ile-107, Ile-111, Ile-112, and Met-131. On the other side of the heme are the other residues: Ile-75, and Ile-142. An examination of the molecular structure shows the strategic placement of each residue. Ile-lll and Ile-112 in the G-helix may be taken as centrally placed. Because of their β-fork structure, these last two side chains make some contact with each other. Through their $C^{\delta 1}$ methyl groups they make contact, respectively, with Ile-28 (B-helix) and Met-131 (H-helix). Ile-28, while not in direct contact, is in communication from the point of view of the packing structure through a common residue, Leu-29, with Met-55 (CD-region). Ile-30, not far from Ile-28, makes direct contact with elements of the D- and E-helices. Ile-111 likewise makes direct contact with elements of the B- and E-helices. Ile-75 (E-helix) makes contact with the border of the heme. Similarly, Ile-142 (H-helix) makes contacts with the F-helix and the heme. Ile-101 (G-helix) makes contact with the H-helix. Ile-107 (G-helix), which could be better studied in a diamagnetic myoglobin form, makes contact with the B- and E-helices in a region whose mobility is attested by the results with the ^{2}H-labeled heme derivative.

The foregoing survey of contacts made by residues whose motions have been assessed to require finite amplitudes and correlation times of the order of 10 ps implies a high average degree of motility within the protein molecule. In view of the characteristics of the ^{13}C-NMR spectra the active motility is the rule not the exception for the probed residues viewed at any instant in time, and will also apply to many other residue types in view of the general ranges of observations of linewidth, T_1 and NOE [38]. It is quite reasonable to expect some of the motions to include those of helices relative to each other by sliding, splaying, or rocking actions. McCammon (et al). [6] pointed out that the motional behavior in the interior of a protein may be viewed either as analogous to liquid behavior or as highly damped harmonic motion more analogous with solid behavior. By comparison with the relaxation behavior of given residues in a small peptide and as probed in the protein the extent of damping is qualitatively obvious. By the same token, the correlation times for the more restricted internal rotational reorientations nevertheless are not greatly increased relative to those surmised from the study of smaller, less encumbered peptides [33-35]. In this connection it is likely that the motion of aliphatic residues within the protein will show shorter correlation times than those of even less hindered external residues bearing highly polar groups [27].

It is interesting that the molecular dynamics treatment [5,6] applied to BPTI produces a similar range in the rotations about the C^α-$C^{\gamma 1}$ bond axis as for the least restricted isoleucine residues listed in Table IV. In BPTI, Ile-18 and Ile-19 are both somewhat exposed to solvent and in 100 ps simulation at 306°K their r.m.s. fluctuations in $\chi_{2,1}$ were 24° and 26°, respectively (J.A. McCammon, personal communication). For comparison a value of 50° in γ_0 in the present treatment of NMR relaxation corresponds to r.m.s. fluctuation of 28°.

Substantial evidence from X-ray crystallography attests to the existence of motions within crystalline proteins [7-10]. Other studies of myoglobins in glasses or glass-like polymers at low temperatures reveal very substantial motility and give indications of the role of the characteristic motional patterns in the functioning of the protein [66]. Since the abutment of one molecule on another in the crystal lattice will restrict or dampen certain potential motional patterns, it is reasonable to expect certain motions to be more pronounced in the dissolved state. To date the analysis of motional behavior from crystallographic measurements over a range of temperatures has been resticted to isotropic treatments but, even so, extensive evidence for internal motion appears well established [7-9]. The information concerning atomic displacements derived from the X-ray measurements may reflect some lattice dampening but it is certain to include the effects of slower displacements than those measurable by NMR in solution in which the rate of overall molecular tumbling presents an effective upper limit to the time scale of observation. Because of these limitations on direct comparison between the methods of X-ray crystallography and NMR of solutions, the recent development of NMR analysis of specifically enriched sites in myoglobin in the crystalline state is particularly promising [29,30].

Acknowledgments

The advice and criticism of Professor Attila Szabo are gratefully acknowledged. The work was supported by National Institutes of Health Grants HL-05556 and HL-14680. This is the 126th paper in a series dealing with coordination complexes and catalytic properties of proteins and related substances.

References

1. C. K. Woodward and B. D. Hilton, *Ann. Rev. Biophys. Bioeng., 8*: 99 (1979).
2. S. W. Englander, D. B. Calhoun, J. J. Englander, N. R. Kallenbach, R. K. H. Liem, E. L. Malin, C. Mandal, and J. R. Rogero, *Biophys. J., 32*:577 (1980).
3. J. R. Lakowicz and G. Weber, *Biochemistry, 12*:4171 (1973).
4. R. F. Chen, H. Edelhoch, and R. F. Steiner, in *Physical Principles and Techniques of Protein Chemistry*, (S. J. Leach, ed.) Academic Press, New York, Part A, 1969, p. 171.
5. M. Karplus and J. A. McCammon, *Crit. Rev. Biochem.*, in press (1980).
6. J. A. McCammon, P. G. Wolynes, and M. Karplus, *Biochemistry, 18*:927 (1979).
7. H. Frauenfelder, G. A. Petsko, and D. Tsernoglou, *Nature (London,* 280:588 (1979).
8. P. J. Artymiuk, C. C. F. Blake, D. E. P. Grace, S. J. Oatley, D. C. Phillips, and M. J. E. Sternberg, *Nature (London), 280:* (1979).
9. H. Frauenfelder and G. A. Petsko, *Biophys. J., 32*:465 (1980).
10. F. R. N. Gurd and T. M. Rothgeb, *Advan. Protein Chem., 33*:73 (1979).
11. D. A. Torchia and D. L. Vanderhart, *J. Mol. Biol., 104*:315 (1976).
12. F. M. Richards, *Carlsberg Res. Commun., 44*:47 (1979).
13. K. Wuthrich, *Nuclear Magnetic Resonance in Biological Research-Peptides and Proteins*, North-Holland Publ., Amsterdam, 1976.
14. K. Wuthrich and G. Wagner, *Trends Biochem. Sci., 3*:227 (1978).

15. R. J. P. Williams, *Proc. Roy. Soc. London, B200*:353 (1978).
16. J. C. Kendrew, *Brookhaven Symp. Biol., 15*:216 (1962).
17. B. Lee and F. M. Richards, *J. Mol. Biol., 55*:379 (1971).
18. T. Takano, *J. Mol. Biol., 110*:569 (1977).
19. R. B. Visscher and F. R. N. Gurd, *J. Biol. Chem., 250*:2238 (1975).
20. J. S. Morrow and F. R. N. Gurd, *Crit. Rev. Biochem., 3*:221, 1975.
21. E. Oldfield, R. S. Norton, and A. Allerhand, *J. Biol. Chem., 250*: 6368 (1975).
22. R. J. Wittebort, Ph.D. Thesis, Indiana University, 1978.
23. R. J. Wittebort and A. Szabo, *J. Chem. Phys., 69*:1722 (1978).
24. R. S. Norton, A. O. Clouse, R. E. Addleman, and A. Allerhand, *J. Am. Chem. Soc., 99*:79 (1976).
25. D. Wallach, *J. Chem. Phys., 47*:5258 (1967).
26. R. E. London and J. Avitabile, *J. Am. Chem. Soc., 100*:7159 (1978).
27. R. J. Wittebort, A. Szabo, and F. R.. N. Gurd, *J. Am. Chem. Soc., 102*:5723 (1980).
28. W. C. Jones, T. M. Rothgeb, and F. R. N. Gurd, *J. Biol. Chem., 251*:7452 (1976).
29. E. Oldfield and T. M. Rothgeb, *J. Am. Chem. Soc., 102*:3635 (1980).
30. T. M. Rothgeb and E. Oldfield, *J. Biol. Chem.* in press.
31. O. Oster, G. W. Neireiter, A. O. Clouse, and F. R. N. Gurd, *J. Biol. Chem., 250*:7990 (1975).
32. G. W. Neireiter, Ph.D. Thesis, Indiana University, 1979.
33. P. Keim, R. A. Vigna, R. C. Marshall, and F. R. N. Gurd, *J. Biol. Chem., 248*:6104 (1973).
34. P. Keim, R. A. Vigna, J. S. Morrow, R. C. Marshall, and F. R. N. Gurd, *J. Biol. Chem., 248*:7811 (1973).
35. P. Keim, R. A. Vigna, A. M. Nigen, J. S. Morrow, and F. R. N. Gurd, *J. Biol. Chem., 249*:4149 (1974).
36. R. A. Bogardt, B. N. Jones, F. E. Dwulet, W. H. Garner, L. D. Lehman, and F. R. N. Gurd, *J. Mol. Evol., 15*:197 (1980).
37. L. H. Botelho, S. H. Friend, J. B. Matthew, L. D. Lehman, G. I. H., Hanania, and F. R. N. Gurd, *Biochemistry, 17*:5197 (1978).
38. R. J. Wittebort, T. M. Rothgeb, A. Szabo, and F. R. N. Gurd, *Proc. Natl. Acad. Sci. USA, 76*:1059 (1979).
39. R. D. DiMarchi, G. W. Neireiter, W. F. Heath, and F. R. N. Gurd, *Biochemistry, 19*:2454 (1980).
40. A. Allerhand, D. Doddrell, V. Glushko, D. W. Cochran, E. Wenkert, P. J. Lawson, and F. R. N. Gurd, *J. Am. Chem. Soc., 93*:544 (1971).
41. V. Glushko, P. J. Lawson, and F. R. N. Gurd, *J. Biol. Chem., 247*:3176 (1972).
42. A. M. Nigen, P. Keim, R. C. Marshall, V. Glushko, P. J. Lawson, and F. R. N. Gurd, *J. Biol. Chem., 248*:3716 (1973).
43. F. M. Richards, *J. Mol. Biol., 82*:1 (1974).
44. T. J. Richmond and F. M. Richards, *J. Mol. Biol., 119*:537 (1978).

45. H. C. Watson, *Progr. Stereochem., 4*:299 (1969).
46. A. B. Edmundson, *Nature (London), 205*:883 (1965).
47. A. E. Romero-Herrera and H. Lehmann, *Proc. Roy. Soc. London, B186*:249 (1974).
48. J. L. Meuth, B. N. Jones, W. H. Garner and F. R. N. Gurd, *Biochemistry, 17*:3429 (1978).
49. F. E. Dwulet, B. N. Jones, L. D. Lehman, and F. R. N. Gurd, *Biochemistry, 16*:873 (1977).
50. D. J. Wilbur, R. S. Norton, A. O. Clouse, R. Addleman, and A. Allerhand, *J. Am. Chem. Soc., 98*:8250 (1976).
51. D. Doddrell, V. Glushko, and A. Allerhand, *J. Chem. Phys., 56*: 3683 (1972).
52. D. E. Woessner and B. S. Snowden, *Adv. Mol. Relax. Proc., 3*:131 (1972).
53. L. Stryer, *Science, 162*:526 (1968).
54. J. Yguerabide, H. F. Epstein, and L. Stryer, *J. Mol. Biol., 51*:573 (1970).
55. S. Otsuka, *Biochem. Biophys. Acta, 214*:233 (1970).
56. I. Morishima and T. Iizuka, *J. Am. Chem. Soc., 96*:7365 (1974).
57. D. A. Ver Ploeg, E. H. Cordes, and F. R. N. Gurd, *J. Biol. Chem., 246*:2725 (1971).
58. W. H. Garner and F. R. N. Gurd, *Biochem. Biophys. Res. Commun., 63*:262 (1975).
59. R. D. DiMarchi, W. H. Garner, C. C. Wang, G. I. H. Hanania, and F. R. N. Gurd, *Biochemistry, 17*:2822 (1978).
60. R. D. DiMarchi, G. W. Neireiter, W. H. Garner, and F. R. N. Gurd, *Biochemistry, 18*:3101 (1979).
61. G. W. Neireiter, R. D. DiMarchi, and F. R. N. Gurd, in *Peptides: Structure and Biological Function*, (E. Gross and J. Meienhofer, eds.), Pierce, Rockville, 1979, p. 621.
62. G. Lipari and A. Szabo, *Biophys. J., 30*:489 (1980).
63. H. Scouloudi, *J. Mol. Biol., 126*:661 (1978).
64. R. A. Bradshaw and F. R. N. Gurd, *J. Biol. Chem., 244*:2167 (1969).
65. F. R. N. Gurd, *Metabolism and Physiological Significance of Lipids*, (R. M. C. Dawson and D. N. Rhodes, eds.), Wiley, New York, 1964, p. 571.
66. R. H. Austin, K. W. Beeson, L. Eisenstein, H. Frauenfelder, and I. C. Gunsalus, *Biochemistry, 14*:5355 (1975).

CHAPTER 2

STUDIES OF CHLOROPHYLL a IN MODEL AND NATURAL MEMBRANE SYSTEMS

Kenneth E. Eigenberg,* William R. Croasmun, and Sunney I. Chan
Division of Chemistry and Chemical Engineering
California Institute of Technology
Pasadena, California

I. INTRODUCTION

In studying biological systems from a chemical point of view, the guiding principle is that there is an important relationship among the structure of the component molecules, the organization of the molecules into structural units, and the function of the system as a whole. Biological membranes, for example, use a relatively limited set of molecules to generate a variety of structures which form organelles with a great diversity in function. One approach to studying these very complex membrane systems is to analyze them in terms of the interactions between the simple building block components. The photosynthetic membrane system is an example of a highly organized system, composed of a relatively limited set of components, whose structure and molecular organization are not very well known though the rudimentary principles of photosynthetic function are fairly well understood.

In plants and some algae, the apparatus for the photosynthetic conversion of light energy into chemical energy is contained within specialized plastic organelles called chloroplasts. Within the outer envelope membrane of chloroplasts is the thylakoid system, a highly organized network of membrane structures which contain a high concentration of pigments.

---

*Present affiliation: Research Department, Monsanto Agricultural Products Co., St. Louis, Missouri

These pigments include two types of chlorophylls, the most abundant of which is chlorophyll a, as well as some accessory carotenoids and phycobilins. Because chlorophyll a is found in nearly all photosynthetic structures, it is considered to be the primary photoreceptor. Photosynthetic harvesting of light energy has traditionally been viewed as a cooperative event in which a group of several hundred chlorophylls function as a photosynthetic unit. Most of the chlorophylls in this unit serve to absorb photon energy and channel it in some nonradiative energy transfer process to a special pair of chlorophylls which act as an energy trap. This special pair is called the reaction center chlorophyll. The chlorophylls transferring energy to the reaction center are referred to as antenna chlorophyll. The bulk of the chlorophyll serves an antenna function, with antenna chlorophylls outnumbering reaction center chlorophylls by several hundred to one.

The structural organization of chlorophyll in the thylakoid membrane is not well understood. Proteins which contain chlorophyll have been isolated from detergent solubilized thylakoid membranes [1], although the apparent amount of protein-associated chlorophyll is variable and usually does not account for all of the *in vivo* chlorophyll. Furthermore, it is possible that part of the chlorophyll is artifactually associated with protein during the detergent solubilization.

We have recently been investigating the possibility that a portion of the chlorophyll a of the thylakoids interacts with the lipids of the thylakoid system to form an array on the surface of the membrane which serves as an antenna network. Indeed, a variety of evidence can be found which suggests that lipids of the thylakoid membrane, in particular monogalactosyldiglyceride (MGD), may have some importance in photosynthesis [2-8]. Figure 1 shows the predominant lipids of the thylakoid system with their approximate relative abundances in parentheses [9]. The glycolipids, monogalactosyldiglyceride (MGD), digalactosyldiglyceride (DGD) and sulfoquinovopyranosyldiglyceride (sulfolipid or SL) comprise 70% of the total lipid mass. Phospholipids, principally phosphatidylglycerol (PG), are only present in small amounts.

An antenna array consisting of lipids interspersed with chlorophylls in the bilayer portion of the thylakoid would have a number of attractive features. First, it allows the antenna to be spread over the surface of the thylakoid and thus be accessible to all of the reaction centers embedded in it. Second, an interspersed array of chlorophyll and lipid molecules could provide ordering of the chlorophylls while separating them at a distance which allows favorable transfer rates. An efficient energy transfer system

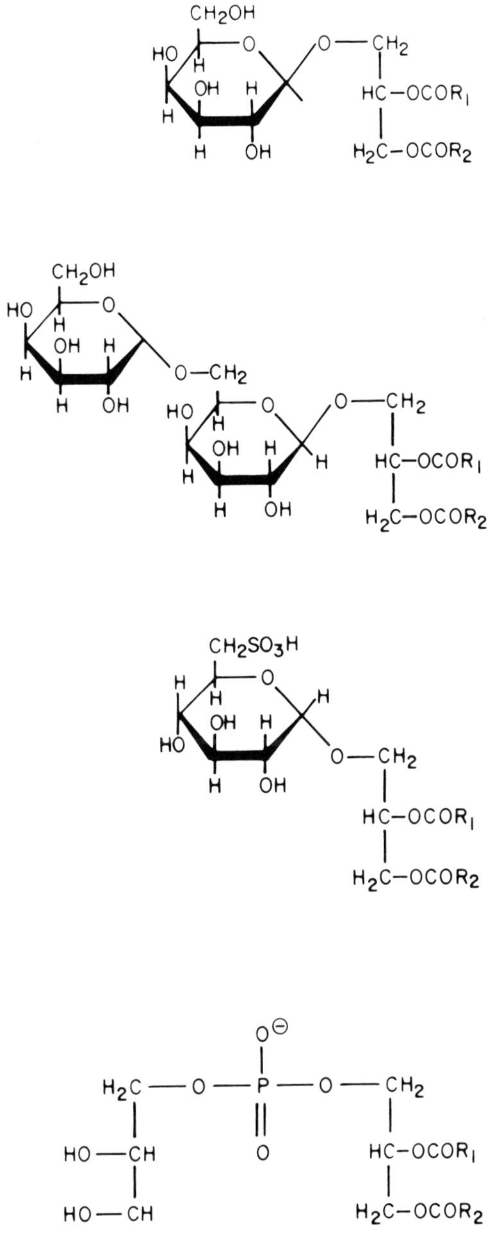

MGD (40%)

DGD (20%)

SL (10%)

PG (20%)

Figure 1. Predominant lipids of the spinach thylakoid membrane with their approximate relative abundances (percent by weight of the total lipids) in parentheses. MGD: monogalactosyldiglyceride, DGD: digalactosyldiglyceride, SL: sulfoquinovopyranosyldiglyceride (plant sulfolipid), PG: phosphatidylglycerol. R_1 and R_2 groups are mostly 16- and 18-carbon highly unsaturated fatty acids.

employing chlorophyll should meet at least three important criteria: a) the chlorophylls should be oriented in a way which provides efficient coupling, b) they should be close enough to allow rapid transfer so as to minimize slower nonradiative relaxation pathways, but c) they should not be close enough to allow trap formation. Calculations [10,11] suggest that two chlorophyll molecules should be at least 10 Å apart to prevent trap formation by orbital overlap. An ordered chlorophyll-lipid array could meet all of these criteria.

Based on chemical considerations, one might expect that chlorophyll should interact with typical membrane lipids. Figure 2 compares the structures and relative dimensions of chlorophyll a and distearoyl phosphatidylcholine (DSPC), a phospholipid with two saturated fatty acid chains similar in length to the phytol chains of chlorophyll. Note that in both molecules there is a well defined interface between the hydrophobic chains and the more polar headgroups. The dual character of chlorophyll, with a hydrophobic chain and a relatively hydrophilic interface region, qualifies it as an amphiphile and it does in fact form monolayers at an air-water interface [12,13]. Chlorophyll by itself does not form bilayer membranes, but in conjunction with other lipids can form black lipid films [14,15], multilayers and small single-walled bilayer vesicles [16-21]. Thus the phytol chain of chlorophyll can apparently serve as a lipophilic anchor to the membrane.

In addition to the phytol chain there are two other structural features of chlorophyll which are potentially important in determining its interactions with other lipid molecules. 1) It is well known that the central magnesium atom is coordinatively unsaturated in the porphyrin and for this reason at least one axial position is always occupied by a ligand donating a pair of electrons [22-24]. This ligand may be for instance an alcohol, ketone, water, or any general Lewis base. An important step in understanding the structural organization of chlorophyll in the thylakoid is to identify this axial ligand to the magnesium. Resonance Raman data [25] indicate that this ligand is not water, nor is it supplied by an adjacent chlorophyll. Thus the axial electron donor is evidently supplied either by lipid or protein groups. 2) The ketone at the carbon-9 position of chlorophyll is important in determining the structure of chlorophyll aggregates in nonpolar solvents [22,23] where the lack of an electron donating solvent forces chlorophyll to satisfy its magnesium coordination requirement by interacting with another chlorophyll molecule through the C_9 ketone. The β-keto ester could also provide a means of binding chlorophyll to the membrane via hydrogen bonding to similar groups on the lipid molecules.

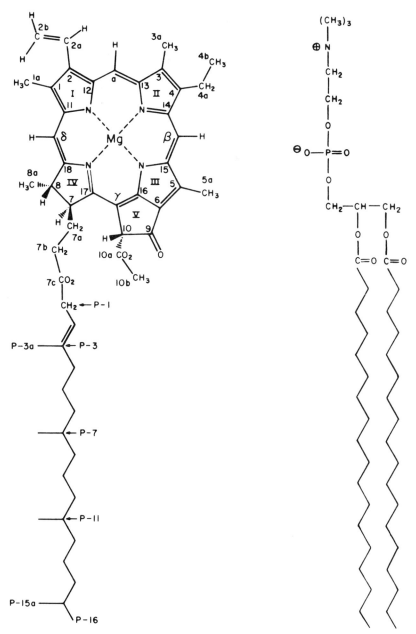

Figure 2.   Chemical structures of chlorophyll a (left) and DSPC, distearoyl phosphatidylcholine (right).

II. STUDIES OF CHLOROPHYLL IN MODEL MEMBRANES

In an effort to understand the interactions of chlorophyll with other lipids in a bilayer matrix, we have studied the bilayer system chlorophyll a/ DSPC by a variety of physical techniques. In particular, differential thermal analysis (DTA) enables us to construct the phase diagram of the system, and NMR studies allow a more complete interpretation of the phase diagram. The well known ring current magnetic anisotropy effect of porphyrins also permits mapping the details of the interaction of chlorophyll a with DSPC.

In these studies chlorophyll a was prepared from spinach extracts by dioxane precipitation [26] and powdered sugar chromatography [27]. Commercial DSPC, which was pure by thin layer chromatography, was used as supplied. Vesicular and multilayer systems were prepared by dissolving chlorophyll a and DSPC in chloroform to ensure adequate mixing, evaporating the solvent under vacuum, and resuspending in H_2O or D_2O. Multilayer systems were prepared by vortexing and heating the aqueous suspension. Vesicle systems were prepared by sonicating the multilayers for 10 minutes while maintaining the sample temperature above the ther-

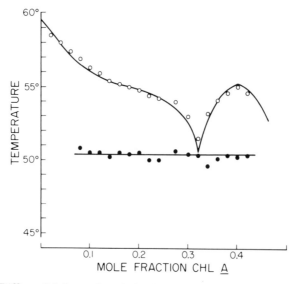

Figure 3.   Differential thermal analysis phase diagram of the chlorophyll a/DSPC bilayer membrane system prepared as an aqueous multilamellar suspension in excess water. Open and closed circles represent points of maximum exothermicity of the observed DTA peaks.

mal phase transition. In this manner, we have been able to prepare vesicles and multilayers which contain up to 45 mole percent chlorophyll a̲.

A. Differential Thermal Analysis Studies

We have examined multilamellar dispersions of chlorophyll a̲ and DSPC by differential thermal analysis on a Dupont 900 DTA instrument. DTA thermograms as a function of chlorophyll composition show two endothermic transitions which coalesce at a eutectic composition near 33 mole percent chlorophyll a̲. At higher chlorophyll concentrations two transitions are again observed. The two transition temperatures (taken as the point of maximum deviation of the recorder trace from the baseline) may be plotted as a function of composition to construct the pseudo-two-component phase diagram of Figure 3. Although the data extended only to 40 mole percent chlorophyll a̲, they appear to comprise a portion of a double-eutectic phase diagram (Figure 4). This diagram implies compound formation between chlorophyll a̲ and DSPC at a compound compo-

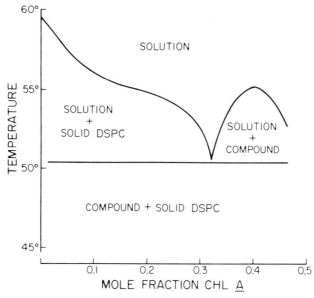

Figure 4. Phase diagram of Figure 3 interpreted in terms of double eutectic phase behavior with accompanying compound formation. Note that only a portion of the double eutectic phase diagram is observed in this system since bilayer structures are not stable with more than about 45 mole percent chlorophyll a.

sition of 40 mole percent. Based on this type of phase behavior the data points can be simulated as a non-ideal binary mixture with a nonzero enthalpy of mixing (K. E. Eigenberg, unpublished results). The agreement between the experimental data and the simulated phase boundary is extremely sensitive to the assumed composition of the compound. The best fit is obtained at a compound composition of 40 mole percent chlorophyll a.

An interesting feature of the phase diagram is that for temperatures below the solidus it predicts an equilibrium between two phases. One phase is essentially pure solid DSPC, while the other is a compound of defined composition formed between DSPC and chlorophyll a. The phase diagram does not, however, specify the nature of the interaction between DSPC and chlorophyll a in the compound phase.

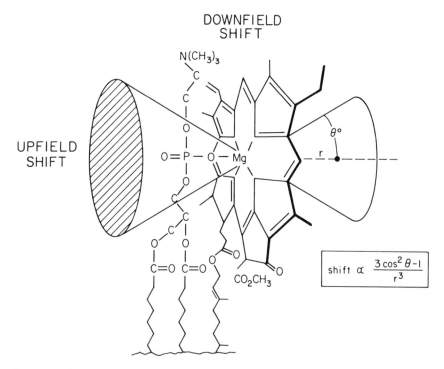

Figure 5. The ring current magnetic anisotropy (or ring current shift effect) of chlorophyll a. Resonance positions of nuclei positioned above the face of the porphyrin macrocycle are shifted upfield by an amount which depends on the distance from, and angle with respect to, the porphyrin plane. Nuclei positioned about the peripheral edge of the porphyrin plane are shifted downfield.

B.   Nuclear Magnetic Resonance Studies

NMR measurements on mixed chlorophyll a/DSPC systems may be used to confirm and extend the observations based on the phase diagram. Chlorophyll-lipid interactions are particularly amenable to study by nuclear magnetic resonance techniques, since the well known ring current magnetic anisotropy effect of the porphyrin macrocycle on nearby molecules can be used to map their distance and orientation with respect to the porphyrin plane. Figure 5 indicates the sign of the ring current shift for a nucleus located at a given position with respect to the chlorophyll macrocycle. This property suggests one possible procedure for deducing the orientation of a neighboring lipid molecule using the ring current shift effect.

In particular this method may be used to verify the existence of the compound phase predicted by the phase diagram. In the phase separated region of the phase diagram below the eutectic temperature, the phospholipids in the two phases should exhibit ^{31}P signals with different chemical shifts, since in the compound the lipid should be closely associated with chlorophyll. In the homogeneous solution region above the liquidus, the phospholipid resonances should show a single solution shift for a ^{31}P nuclei.

1. ^{31}P NMR

The results of ^{31}P NMR experiments with sonicated chlorophyll a/DSPC (1:4) vesicles verify these predictions from the phase diagram. Spectra obtained on a Varian XL-100 at two temperatures are shown in Figure 6. Above the upper transition temperature a single phospholipid resonance is obtained, while below the eutectic temperature two phospholipid peaks are observed. One of the two peaks has a chemical shift nearly identical to that of the single peak obtained at high temperature, while the new peak is shifted 5.8 ppm upfield. The observation of two peaks confirms that phase separation does indeed occur at temperatures below the solidus.

In addition, the magnitude of the phosphorous shift is quite informative. We assume that the only source of shift arises from the ring current anisotropy, and use a previously derived empirical expression for the magnitude of the ring current shift for nuclei located at various distances and orientations with respect to the porphyrin plane [28]. If we presuppose that the phosphorous of DSPC is centered above the plane of the porphyrin then the magnitude of the observed shift corresponds to a magnesium

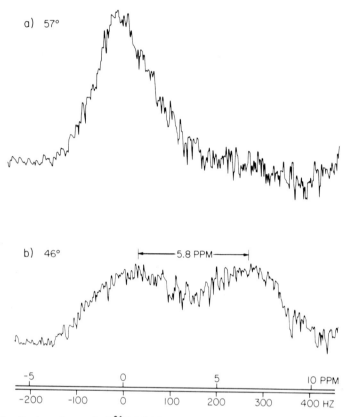

Figure 6. Proton decoupled ^{31}P-NMR spectra at 40.5 MHz of sonicated chlorophyll a/DSPC (1:4) single-walled bilayer vesicles at 57° (top) and 46° (bottom). At 57° the membranes are in the solution region of the phase diagram. At 46° the phase diagram predicts phase separation into solid DSPC and compound phases.

to phosphorous distance of 3.4 Angstroms. This is quite consistent with an MG·· O-P coordination bond distance. Any other geometry would predict a magnesium to phosphorous distance which is unreasonably short. It may be that the obligatory coordination requirement of the chlorophyll a central magnesium atom is satisfied by the phosphate of DSPC in this system.

2. ^{13}C-NMR

Other nuclei contiguous with phosphorous in the DSPC headgroup should also show ring current shifts. Unfortunately, in ^{13}C spectra of vesicles

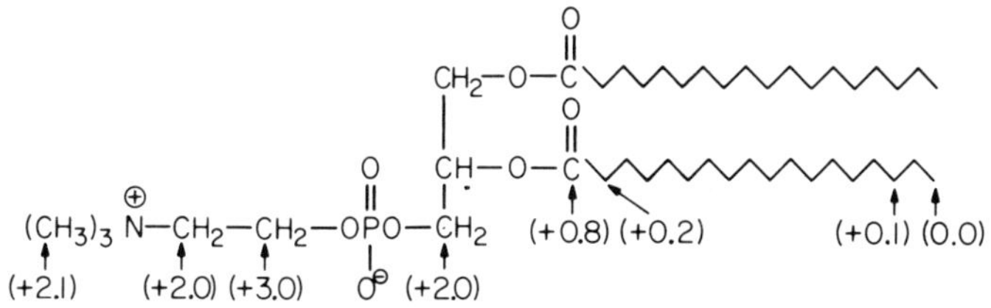

Figure 7. The chemical shift differences (in ppm) between equimolar chlorophyll a/DSPC in CCl_4 and DSPC alone in CCl_4 for various carbons of DSPC.

composed of chlorophyll a and DSPC, the lipid resonances are too broad to resolve shifts of this magnitude. Accordingly, we have investigated the interaction between chlorophyll a and DSPC in CCl_4 solution where the ^{13}C resonance widths are narrower. In Figure 7 the chemical shift differences (in ppm) between equimolar chlorophyll a/DSPC in CCl_4 and DSPC alone in CCl_4 are shown for various carbons of the lipid. The largest shifts are observed in the headgroup region and the size of the shift decreases with distance from the phosphate. Since the ring current shift increases toward and is largest near the phosphorous it appears that the phosphate moiety is located near the center of the porphyrin plane, directly above the magnesium. This observation is consistent with the conclusion that chlorophyll a interacts with DSPC via coordination of the central magnesium with phosphate.

3. ^1H-NMR

We have undertaken ^1H-NMR experiments as a function of temperature at two frequencies, 100 and 360 MHz, to verify the overall features of the phase diagram. These measurements were made on a Varian XL-100 and the Bruker HXS-360 spectrometer at the Stanford Magnetic Resonance Laboratory. The ^1H-NMR spectra of sonicated chlorophyll a/DSPC (1:4) vesicles at both fields show only a single choline methyl resonance over a temperature range encompassing all regions of the phase diagram. For the following reasons, this observation suggests that below the liquidus the chemical shift difference between the DSPC cholines in the two phases is small: 1) If the single observed resonance is a superposition of two nonexchanging resonances, then the shift difference between them must be less than the observed choline resonance linewidth (about 50 Hz). 2) Suppose on the other hand that the single resonance line results from two pools of lipids in fast exchange on the timescale of the ^{1}H experiment. The ^{31}P experiment indicates that the exchange rate is less than the observed splitting of 230 Hz. If the ^{1}H experiment is indeed in the fast exchange regime, then the shift difference between the ^{1}H resonances should be significantly less than 230 Hz, and the exchange rate must be between the timescales set by the ^{1}H and ^{31}P chemical shift differences. Assuming that the exchange rate is determined by the rate of lateral diffusion of the lipid, then an exchange rate of 100 Hz and a diffusion coefficient of 10^{-10} cm^2/ sec would correspond to a reasonable domain size of 10^4 square Angstroms. Dispersion versus absorption (DISPA) plots of the choline methyl ^{1}H resonance below the liquidus indicate that the lineshape does indeed have contributions from two or more components with different linewidths but nearly identical chemical shift [29]. Thus, we may reject the suggestion that the resonance from one of the lipid pools is so broad that it does not contribute to the observed lineshape. The DISPA data does not permit a conclusion as to whether the various components are exchanging on the timescale of the experiment.

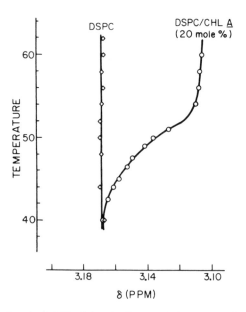

Figure 8.   The chemical shift of the choline methyl protons of DSPC in DSPC and chlorophyll a/DSPC (1:4) sonicated vesicles as a function of temperature. Data were obtained at 360 MHz using an external TMS reference and corrected for changes in solvent bulk susceptibility with temperature.

Both the chemical shifts and the linewidths of the various lipid proton resonances in mixed chlorophyll a/DSPC vesicles are temperature dependent. The shift of the choline methyl protons of DSPC in sonicated DSPC and sonicated chlorophyll a/DSPC (1:4) vesicles are compared in Figure 8. (These data have been corrected for the change in bulk susceptibility with temperature). At low temperatures the shift of the choline methyl protons in chlorophyll a/DSPC vesicles is nearly the same as that for DSPC vesicles without chlorophyll a. As the temperature is raised, a small upfield shift is observed as a solution of DSPC and chlorophyll a is formed. The temperature at which the shift begins is approximately the eutectic temperature. We interpret this small shift in the solution region in terms of the solution shift normally observed for molecules dissolved in aromatic solvents.

Proton linewidths also show a temperature dependence. Figure 9 shows this dependence for two lipid resonances of chlorophyll a/DSPC (1:4)

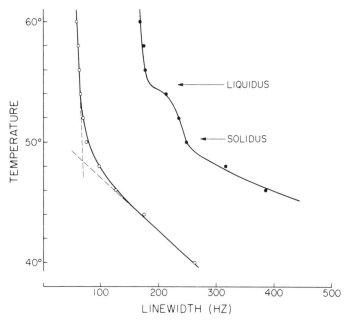

Figure 9. Linewidths at half height of the choline methyl (open circles, left) and bulk fatty acid methylene (closed circles, right) lipid resonances from chlorophyll a/DSPC (1:4) vesicles as a function of temperature. The liquidus and solidus temperatures at this composition are indicated by arrows. These data were obtained from spectra at 360 MHz.

vesicles. There is an abrupt change in the slope of the dependence for the choline methyl resonances at about 49°C, corresponding approximately to the solidus of the phase diagram. Methylenes become broadened at a somewhat higher temperature, corresponding to the liquidus of the phase diagram, with a further break at the solidus. These changes in the slope of the linewidth versus temperature occur upon formation or elimination of a phase at a boundary of the phase diagram and correspond to changes in the overall motional state of the lipids.

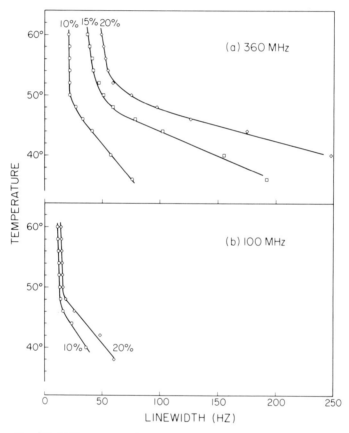

Figure 10. Field/frequency dependence of the choline methyl resonance linewidths in chlorophyll a/DSPC sonicated vesicles. a) Data as a function of temperature for 10, 15, and 20 mole percent chlorophyll a at 360 MHz (84.56 Kilogauss). b) Data for 10 and 15 mole percent chlorophyll at 100 MHz (23.49 Kilogauss).

In addition to their temperature dependence, proton linewidths for the choline methyl groups also vary with the field/frequency used in these experiments (Figure 10). Using ^{1}H-NMR data at 100 MHz and 360 MHz, we find that the linewidths may be resolved into two contributions, one of which is field independent while the other depends on the square of the static magnetic field. The magnitude of the field independent part of the linewidth is nearly independent of the chlorophyll concentration, while that of the field dependent term depends strongly on chlorophyll content. The field dependent contribution to the linewidth may be interpreted in terms of a chemical shift anisotropy relaxation mechanism. Since the field/ frequency dependent contribution to the linewidth depends on chlorophyll concentration and is absent for pure DSPC vesicles, the chemical shift anisotropy of the choline evidently arises from its proximity to the porphyrin ring. This chemical shift anisotropy is modulated by vesicle tumbling. In the limit $\omega_0 \tau_c >> 1$ we have [30]

$$\frac{1}{T_2} = \frac{1}{10} \gamma^2 H_0^2 (\Delta\sigma)^2 \tau_c.$$

Using the Stokes relationship to relate the correlation time of vesicle tumbling to vesicle radius, we find that the observed contribution of the field dependent mechanism to the linewidth at temperatures below the solidus may be accounted for assuming a vesicle radius of 500 Angstroms and a chemical shift anisotropy $\Delta\sigma$ of approximately 2 ppm. To our knowledge our results here represent the first evidence for a chemical shift anisotropy contribution to a proton nuclear spin relaxation, albeit in a rather atypical situation.

III. CHLOROPHYLL IN NATURAL MEMBRANES

From the studies of chlorophyll in model bilayer membranes just discussed it appears that chlorophyll interacts in a very specific manner with the lipids in a phospholipid bilayer matrix. We now wish to determine whether or not similar interactions occur in natural photosynthetic membranes. To ascertain this point we have used NMR to study the motional state of chlorophyll in the thylakoid membrane itself. The lateral mobility and internal flexibility of chlorophyll will be influenced by the way in which it is bound to the membrane and, thus, NMR linewidths may be used to infer the structural organization of chlorophyll in the membrane.

We have recorded ^{13}C-NMR spectra of intact thylakoid membranes from spinach. These spectra exhibit well-resolved resonances which can be assigned to specific membrane components. The linewidths and apparent intensities of these resonances have allowed us to reach some limited conclusions concerning the organization of chlorophyll in the membrane. In particular the data suggest that there is indeed a pool of chlorophyll in the photosynthetic thylakoid membrane associated with membrane lipids.

For these studies thylakoid membranes were obtained from spinach by procedures which do not alter their native structure. Whole chloroplasts were harvested from the leaves of fresh spinach by homogenization in isotonic sucrose buffer and centrifugation to remove cell debris. Thylakoid membranes were then isolated from the intact chloroplasts by osmotic lysis of the double outer envelope membranes in a hypotonic medium [9]. The thylakoids were then pelleted by centrifugation and resuspended several times to effect complete separation of the thylakoid and envelope membrane fractions. All buffer media contained cations which prevent the dissociation and swelling of the thylakoid grana [31]. The optical spectrum of thylakoid membranes isolated in this manner was found to be essentially indistinguishable from that of whole chloroplasts.

Proton-decoupled Fourier transform ^{13}C spectra at 90.5 MHz of the resulting thylakoid preparation were obtain at 25°C on a Bruker HXS-360 spectrometer at the Stanford Magnetic Resonance Laboratory within 24 hours of sample preparation. Transients were collected every 2.5 seconds using 16 K data points and a spectral width of 20 KHz.

The resulting ^{13}C-NMR spectrum, Figure 11, shows many distinct resonances which may be identified by comparison with previous spectra of chlorophyll a [32,33] and other thylakoid lipids [34-36]. The assignments of these resonances are facilitated by the homogeneity of the galactolipid hydrocarbon chains (16:3 and 18:3 fatty acids comprise 90% of the total), [37,38], and by the fact that porphyrin resonances are not observed because of the rigidity of the porphyrin macrocycle and the additional motional restriction imposed by the binding of chlorophyll to the membrane. The resonance assignments, shown in Figures 12a, 12b, and 12c, indicate that virtually all of the lines in the high resolution spectrum can be assigned either to galactolipid or to phytol chains of chlorophyll. Resonances from membrane proteins are notably absent from the spectrum.

The relative intensities of the various galactolipid resonances are consistent with their mole fractions in the membrane, although the intensities of the chlorophyll resonances relative to similar resonances of the lipids are

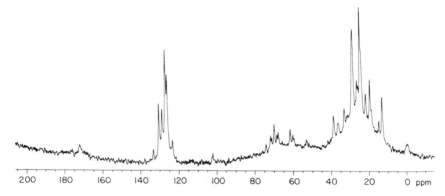

Figure 11. Proton-decoupled natural abundance 90.5 MHz ^{13}C Fourier transform NMR spectrum of isolated spinach thylakoid membranes of 25°C. The sample consisted of a loosely packed pellet of thylakoid membranes in D_2O in a 10 mm tube. A total of 26, 875 transients were accumulated and Fourier transformed to yield the above spectrum. The chemical shift scale is in parts per million relative to tetramethylsilane.

somewhat less than might be expected. Comparison of the spectral intensities of thylakoid chlorophyll resonances with spectral intensities of chlorophyll a — phospholipid model bilayer systems under equivalent experimental conditions indicates that only 30 ± 10% of the total chlorophyll complement of the thylakoid membrane is observed in the high resolution spectrum.

The absence of protein resonances in the thylakoid ^{13}C-NMR spectrum is consistent with previous ^{13}C studies of other biological membranes where the high resolution spectrum is observed to arise from lipids only [39]. ^{13}C relaxation mechanisms in large molecules are intramolecular and therefore related to internal segmental motions [40]. Thus protein resonances are not observed (i.e. are broad) because of incomplete motional averaging resulting from restricted internal motion or long motional correlation times. Conversely, the relatively narrow phytol resonances of the observed chlorophyll must indicate more complete motional averaging. We may therefore conclude that the 30% pool of chlorophyll observed in the high resolution ^{13}C spectrum has a motional state which is much different than protein, but approximately the same as that of the lipid portion of the membrane. Thus our results argue against the notion that the chlorophyll observed here is embedded in membrane protein. More likely, this chlorophyll is contained in the bilayer portion of the membrane

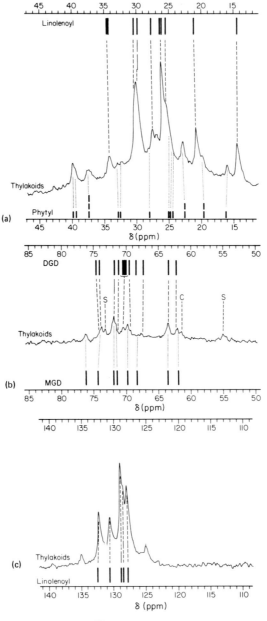

Figure 12. Assignments of the ^{13}C-NMR spectrum from spinach thylakoids. Selected regions of Figure 11 are expanded for ease of comparison. a) Saturated carbon region (10-45 ppm). Positions of phytol and linolenic fatty acid resonances are indicated by vertical bars. b) Galactolipid headgroup and glycerol backbone region (50-85 ppm). Positions of MGD and DGD resonances are indicated by the bars. The letters S and C indicate peaks assignable to sulfolipid (S) and chlorophyll (C). c) Unsaturated carbon region (110-140 ppm). Positions of linolenic acid resonances are again indicated by bars. Resonances assigned but not shown: galactosyl C-1 of MGD (104.8 ppm), fatty acid carbonyls (172 ppm).

or perhaps bound at the periphery of membrane protein. In either of these two cases, the phytol chains would have sufficient freedom of motion to yield the linewidths observed in the ^{13}C spectrum.

In view of much good evidence for the location of reaction center chlorophyll in protein complexes and for the heterogeneity of spectral classes of chlorophyll, we consider it likely that there are several pools of chlorophyll in the thylakoid membrane. Our conclusions from the ^{13}C spectrum of thylakoids, as well as other evidence in the literature, suggest that at least one of these pools of chlorophyll involves membrane lipid.

IV. SUMMARY

Nuclear magnetic resonance measurements as a function of temperature have been used to investigate the phase behavior, motional state and molecular interactions of chlorophyll a with other membrane lipids in model and natural membrane systems. In the model systems, differential thermal analysis data suggest that mixed chlorophyll a/DSPC model membranes have a double eutectic phase diagram exhibiting compound formation at about 40 mole % chlorophyll a. Such a phase diagram predicts an equilibrium between free solid DSPC and compound at temperatures below the solidus. ^{31}P NMR spectra of mixed chlorophyll a/DSPC vesicles confirm that phase separation occurs at low temperatures and suggest along with ^{13}C data that the axial coordination requirement of the chlorophyll magnesium may be met by the phosphate of the lipid. Finally, the temperature dependence of ^{1}H NMR linewidths and chemical shifts reflects changes in the motional state of the lipid and its proximity to chlorophyll as the boundaries of the phase diagram are traversed. The choline proton linewidths were found to be field dependent as well as chlorophyll concentration dependent. These observations may be interpreted in terms of a contribution to relaxation from a chemical shift anisotropy mechanism, the anisotropy originating from the proximity of the lipid headgroup to the porphyrin ring in the compound phase.

The compound provides a lipid-containing chlorophyll phase of defined composition. Such a phase could provide ordering of chlorophylls and separation of chlorophylls at a distance optimal for efficient energy transfer. Thus it is an attractive model for a photosynthetic antenna in vivo.

To investigate the relevance of the data from model systems to photosynthetic systems in vivo, it is first necessary to verify the existence of lipid-associated chlorophyll in the thylakoid membrane. To this end we have obtained the ^{13}C spectrum of native thylakoid membranes. A number of well-resolved lines are obtained, which may be assigned to the headgroup and hydrocarbon chains of thylakoid glycolipids and to the phytol chain of chlorophyll a. Protein resonances are notably absent from the spectrum. The observation of well-resolved chlorophyll resonances in the absence of protein resonances indicates that the observed chlorophyll has a motional state very different than that of membrane protein, and suggests that this pool of chlorophyll is associated with the lipid portion of the thylakoid or possibly located at the periphery of a membrane protein, rather than being bound in the hydrophobic interior of a protein.

Acknowledgments

This work was supported by United States Public Health Service Grant GM-22432 from the National Institute of General Medical Sciences. KEE and WRC were supported during the time of this work by NIH National Research Service Awards GM-07616 and GM-01262 from the National Institute of General Medical Sciences. Several of the experiments were carried out at the Stanford Magnetic Resonance Laboratory which is supported by NSF Grant GP-23633 and NIH Grant RR-00711. This is contribution No. 6216 from the Division of Chemistry and Chemical Engineering, California Institute of Technology.

References

1. J. P. Thornber, J. P. Markwell, and S. Reinman, *Photochem. Photobiol.,* *29*:1205 (1979).
2. J. C. Beck and R. P. Levin, *Biochim. Biophys. Acta, 489*:360 (1977).
3. K. P. Heise and G. Jacobi, *Planta, 111*:137 (1973).
4. P. G. Roughan and N. K. Boardman, *Plant Physiol., 50*:31 (1972).
5. A. Tremolieres and M. Lepage, *Plant Physiol., 47*:329 (1971).
6. E. S. Bamberger and R. B. Park, *Plant Physiol., 41*:1591 (1966).
7. Z. Krupa and T. Baszynski, *Biochim. Biophys. Acta, 408*:26 (1975).
8. L. K. Ostrovskaya, S. M. Kochubei, and T. M. Shadchina, *Biokhimiya, 40*:169 (1975).
9. H. Hashimoto and S. Murakami, *Plant Cell Physiol., 16*:895 (1975).
10. G. S. Beddard and G. Porter, *Nature, 260*:366 (1976).
11. G. S. Beddard, S. E. Carlin, and G. Porter, *Chem. Phys. Lett., 43*:27 (1976).
12. B. Ke, in *The Chlorophylls) (L. P. Vernon and G. R. Seely, eds.) Academic Press, New York, 1966, p. 253.*
13. *G. L. Gaines, W. D. Bellamy, and A. G. Tweet, J. Chem. Phys., 41*:538 (1964).

14. A. Steinemann, N. Alamuti, W. Brodman, O. Marschall, and P. Läuger, *J. Membrane Biol., 4*:284 (1971).
15. H. P. Ting, W. A. Huemueller, S. Lalitha, A. L. Diana, and H. T. Tien, *Biochim. Biophys. Acta, 163*:439 (1968).
16. K. Colbow, *Biochim. Biophys. Acta, 314*:320 (1973).
17. A. Mehreteab and G. Strauss, *Photochem. Photobiol., 28*:369 (1978).
18. E. Ritt and D. Walz, *J. Membrane Biol., 27*:141 (1976).
19. H. Dijkmans, R. M. Leblanc, F. Cogniaux, and J. Aghion, *Photochem. Photobiol., 29*:367 (1979).
20. F. Podo, J. E. Cain, and J. K. Blasie, *Biochim. Biophys. Acta, 419*:19 (1976).
21. W. Oettmeir, J. R. Norris, and J. J. Katz, *Biochem. Biophys. Res. Commun., 71*:445 (1976).
22. J. J. Katz, J. R. Norris, and L. Shipman, *Brookhaven Symp. Biol. 28th*, 16 (1976).
23. J. J. Katz, *Inorg. Biochem., 2*:1022 (1973).
24. J. J. Katz, *Dev. Appl. Spec., 6*:201 (1968).
25. M.Lutz, *Biochim. Biophys. Acta, 460*:408 (1977).
26. K. Iriyama, N. Ogura, and A. Takamiya, *J. Biochem., 76*:901 (1974).
27. H. H. Strain, M. R. Thomas, H. L. Crespi, M. I. Blake, and J. J. Katz, *Ann. New York Acad. Sci., 84*:617 (1960).
28. R. G. Shulman, K. Wüthrich, T. Yamane, D. J. Patel, and W. E. Blumberg, *J. Mol. Biol., 53*:143 (1970).
29. A. G. Marshall and D. C. Roe, *Analyt. Chem., 50*:756 (1978).
30. A. Abragam, *The Principles of Nuclear Magnetism*, Clarendon, Oxford, 1961, p. 316.
31. S. Murakami and L. Packer, *Arch. Biochem. Biophys., 146*:337 (1971).
32. R. A. Goodman, E. Oldfield, and A. Allerhand, *J. Am. Chem. Soc., 95*:7553 (1973).
33. S. G. Boxer, G. L. Closs, and J. J. Katz, *J. Am. Chem. Soc., 96*:7058 (1974).
34. S. R. Johns, D. R. Leslie, R. I. Willing, and D. G. Bishop, *Aus. J. Chem., 30*:823 (1977).
35. S. R. Johns, D. R. Leslie, R. I. Willing, and D. G. Bishop, *Aus. J. Chem., 31*:65 (1978).
36. S. R. Johns, D. R. Leslie, R. I. Willing, and D. G. Bishop, *Aus. J. Chem., 30*:813 (1977).
37. A. T. James and B. W. Nichols, *Nature, 210*:372 (1966).
38. C. F. Allen and P. Good, *Methods Enz., 23*:523 (1971).
39. K. M. Keough, E. Oldfield, D. Chapman, and P. Beynon, *Chem. Phys. Lipids, 10*:37 (1973).
40. A. Allerhand, D. Doddrell, and R. Komoroski, *J. Chem. Phys., 55*:189 (1971).

CHAPTER 3

25Mg NMR APPLICATIONS TO PROBLEMS IN BIOPHYSICAL CHEMISTRY

Deni M. Rose*, P.A. Tovo†, and Robert G. Bryant
Department of Chemistry
University of Minnesota
Minneapolis, Minnesota

M. Louise Bleam‡ and M. Thomas Record, Jr.
Department of Chemistry
University of Wisconsin
Madison, Wisconsin

I. INTRODUCTION

The alkaline earth metal ions are crucial inorganic cofactors for a large number of enzyme catalyzed reactions that in turn are central to life processes [1]. In addition to the highly specific interactions usually associated with enzyme catalysis and well known for low molecular weight compounds, the alkaline earth ions may have a general function as a consequence of their charge in the presence of anionic polyelectrolytes often present in living materials. For example, the response of DNA melting curves to divalent metal ions suggests that group IIA ions may be structural effectors simply by virtue of their electric charge [2].

Magnesium ion is well known to associate with anionic ligands in aqueous solutions. The association constant expressed in concentration units of ($\ell \cdot mole^{-1}$) is dependent on ionic strength but is usually reported to

---

*Present affiliation: Engineering Research Center, Western Electric Co., Princeton, New Jersey.

†Present affiliation: Honeywell Corporation, Minneapolis, Minnesota.

‡Present affiliation: Department of Chemistry, Central College, Pella, Iowa.

be greater than 10^2 for representative phosphate systems [3]. A somewhat surprising aspect of magnesium chemistry is its inertness to ligand exchange compared with alkali metals and calcium ions [4]. Water exchange lifetimes in the magnesium ion first coordination sphere are reported to be on the order of tenths to hundredths of msec [5]. Lifetimes of magnesium ion coordinated to phosphate are reported to be in the range from msec to .1 msec [6]. Although chemical exchange may make important contributions to magnesium relaxation in phosphate systems, the fast exchange conditions so often associated with relaxation of nuclei such as sodium and chlorine may fail for the magnesium case.

The interaction of simple ions such as magnesium ion with polyelectrolytes like DNA may be treated from two points of view that we will consider as extremes. One may treat the binding of the metal ion as an interaction with specific sites on the macromolecule using a mass action formulation that depends on the equilibrium constants for alkaline earth ion phosphate interactions. On the other hand a weak but important loose association in addition to or instead of site interactions is expected based on a consideration of the electrostatics of the charged linear polyelectrolyte problem [7]. Depending on relative counterion and polyion concentrations, the mathematical consequences of such an electrostatic interaction can be much the same as those for a mass action formulation and some care must be used to assess the relative importance of each. ^{23}Na NMR has been used successfully to demonstrate the importance of the electrostatic condensation of sodium ions into the domain adjacent to a DNA molecule [8]. Such interactions will be called domain binding, and are characterized by the retention of a full first hydration sphere by the counterion. In contrast we assume that counterion interactions with particular residues on the polyelectrolyte involve the loss of one or more water molecules from the counterion's first coordination sphere. This latter type of interaction will be referred to as site binding. The present research was motivated by a desire to test the importance of these two types of interaction potentially possible for the alkaline earth ions.

^{25}Mg NMR was chosen for the investigation primarily because magnesium ion is found at reasonable concentrations in many physiological environments where calcium appears to be more often buffered at significantly lower concentrations. In addition direct observation of the metal ion eliminates any difficulties often associated with indirect observations of some probe ion such as Co(II) and Mn(II). Due to inherent difficulties with sensitivity and low resonant frequency, ^{25}Mg NMR has only recently become a readily available technique for studying cation behavior in biological systems. The earliest applications of ^{25}Mg NMR to biological problems were those of Magnuson and Bothner-By [9] and Bryant [10], who studied the linebroadening effect of Mg^{+2} complexation to various carboxylic acids and biologically interesting phosphates. The wider availability of Fourier transform techniques and higher magnetic fields has simplified observation of the ^{25}Mg resonance at biologically relevant concentrations. The ^{25}Mg isotope is relatively inexpensive to obtain at higher enrichments and it is now possible to obtain spectra with reasonable sensitivity in a matter of minutes at concentrations down to the millimolar range. A number of recent studies have utilized this capability to study the binding of magnesium to various proteins, peptides, and nucleic acids [11-15].

The present discussion will include a summary of fundamental magnesium relaxation parameters since a complete investigation has not appeared. Representative results of Mg^{+2} complexation studies in low molecular weight phosphate systems will be presented, as well as some preliminary results on Mg^{+2} interactions with DNA.

II. EXPERIMENTAL

^{25}Mg NMR spectra were accumulated in a 1.4 T magnetic field provided by a field frequency locked Varian 12-inch electromagnet. An 18 mm x 18 mm single coil configuration was used to contain 15 mm tubes housed in a stainless steel probe body to minimize ring-down transients. The probe was driven by an ENI 10 watt amplifier and the 90 degree pulse width ranged from 42 to 150 microsec depending on the details of the probe impedence matching circuitry used. The spectrometer operated at 3.45 MHz. Vari-L r.f. gates driven by a Nicolet NMR-80 data system controlled transmitter r.f. from a Hewlett-Packard 8660B frequency synthesizer. Single phase detection was used in a receiver constructed in this laboratory. A Rockland audio filter was employed in front of the Nicolet mainframe. The effective ring down time of the receiver assembly in this configuration was shorter than 500 microsec when 20,000 transients were averaged.

The enriched magnesium isotope was obtained as the oxide from Union Carbide facilities at Oak Ridge, Tennessee, dissolved in metal free hydrochloric acid, and the solid chloride recovered by vacuum evaporation. Solutions of the desired magnesium chloride concentration were prepared by dissolving the solid in deionized water. Concentrations were determined gravimetrically or spectrophotometrically [16]. Calf thymus DNA was obtained from Worthington Company and prepared as previously described [8].

III. RESULTS AND DISCUSSION

Two ²⁵Mg NMR spectra, shown in Fig. 1, demonstrate several features of alkaline earth NMR spectroscopy. 1) For aqueous solutions of magnesium electrolytes the NMR line shape is Lorentzian as anticipated for cases where all observed nuclei experience extreme narrowing conditions [17]. 2) For a more complicated system such as DNA solution, a simple Lorentzian line shape is not observed. 3) The signal to noise ratio is more than adequate for studies in reasonable lengths of time at concentrations that approach physiologically sensible levels.

Magnesium ion is well known to be one of the more substitutionally inert nontransition elements [18]. Since the solvent lifetimes in the magnesium first coordination sphere are expected to be long compared with the reciprocal of the Larmor frequency, a significant difference between longitudinal and transverse relaxation times will result if a significant magnetic interaction is modulated by the exchange reaction. The data of Fig. 2, however, demonstrate that longitudinal and transverse relaxation rates are equal in simple magnesium chloride solutions. Studies as a function of solvent isotope composition demonstrate that there is no de-

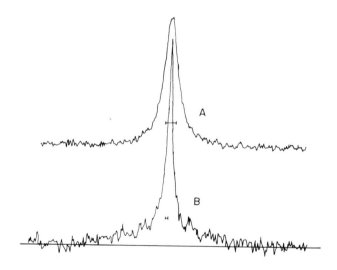

Figure 1. A. ²⁵Mg NMR spectrum of 2.89 molal magnesium acetate recorded at 3.45 MHz. B. ²⁵Mg NMR spectrum of 0.114 M MgCl₂ approximately 8.3 mM in unsonicated calf thymus DNA phosphate. The scale mark for each spectrum represents 50 Hz.

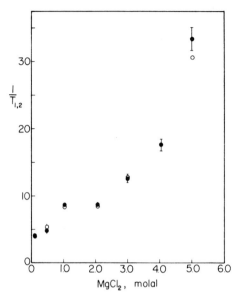

Figure 2. 25Mg NMR relaxation rates at 3.45 MHz as a function of $MgCl_2$ concentration. Longitudinal relaxation rates shown as solid circles were measured by the inversion recovery method. Transverse relaxation rates shown as open circles were measured using the Meiboom-Gill modification of the Carr-Purcell pulse sequence.

tectable relaxation caused by direct dipole-dipole interactions with solvent protons or scalar relaxation of either the first or second kind [17] caused by coupling to solvent deuterons or 17O nuclei. Hence, 25Mg NMR relaxation is dominated by the nuclear electric quadrupole interaction.

The quadrupole relaxation mechanism in general and magnesium resonances in particular are known to respond to changes in ligation of the metal ion because of changes in the electric field gradient at the magnesium nucleus, changes in the correlation time for the reorientation of the field gradient, or both [9-15,19]. In addition chemical exchange events may be crucial. The importance of chemical exchange as a potentially dominant contribution to 25Mg NMR relaxation in macromolecule solutions was emphasized some time ago [10]. Work is presently in progress to survey the exchange rates of magnesium ion with the common biochemical functional groups. The temperature dependence for representative phosphate systems is shown in Fig. 3. The solid lines drawn through the data represent a fit to the chemical exchange model summarized by Swift and Connick [20]. Clearly the temperature dependences of the magnesium

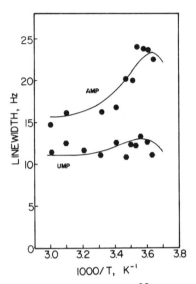

Figure 3. The temperature dependence of the ^{25}Mg NMR linewidth in aqueous adenosine monophosphate and uridine monophosphate solutions. Each sample was 0.019 M in nucleotide and 0.093 M in ^{25}MgCl$_2$ at pH 8. Solid lines through the data represent fits to the chemical exchange model of Swift and Connick and include corrections for the temperature dependence of the magnesium-phosphate association constants.

relaxation rates in the presence of AMP and UMP are different; both imply a contribution of the exchange rate to the relaxation rates. The parameters required to fit the present data for these nucleotides require a significant chemical shift on binding, activation energies of 12-13 kcal/mole and rate constants of 3 x 10^3 sec^{-1} at 298 K. In addition there appears to be a small but systematic difference between purine and pyrimidine nucleotide exchange parameters, chemical shifts, and relaxation parameters required in the fit [21]. The curves shown in Fig. 3 were calculated including a correction for the temperature dependence of the magnesium-phosphate association constants. We anticipate that such corrections will be required generally in analysis of alkaline earth-ligand interactions at the lower concentrations appropriate to physiological levels. In summary, these data demonstrate that chemical exchange effects may generally complicate analysis of magnesium NMR spectra.

In a high molecular weight polyelectrolyte such as DNA, several types of counterion-polyion interactions may be important. In aqueous solutions of DNA we anticipate that the observed relaxation behavior of ^{25}Mg^{+2}

will be influenced by the lifetimes and relaxation rates of magnesium ions in a number of distinct environments. These may include more than one type of "bound" interaction as defined previously and shown schematically in Fig. 4. The ^{23}Na NMR data for DNA solutions [22] may guide our analysis of the ^{25}Mg data. For sodium ion, specific site interactions are minimal or absent. In the magnesium case, however, exchange of the metal ion with phosphate as well as other sites may contribute an additional broadening. If the exchange between the bulk magnesium pool and nonspecifically bound or domain bound regions is rapid, it will be difficult to separate and quantitate the relative contributions from each interaction to relaxation. Temporarily neglecting the exchange contributions, the aqueous magnesium ion relaxation rates in DNA free solutions are about half those of sodium at equivalent concentrations. Thus the linewidth for ^{25}Mg in the domain region of DNA should be half that for sodium ion or about 30 Hz [8,22]. The data in Fig. 1 are not even approximately consistent with this analysis. We suggest that a major contribution to magnesium relaxation in DNA solutions arises from site specific interactions. It is not

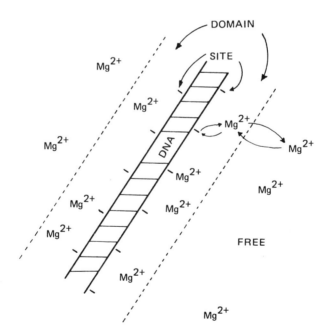

Figure 4. Schematic representation of the modes of interaction between magnesium ion and DNA.

clear, however, that the system may be described as a limiting two site situation (bound and free magnesium ions) for several reasons: 1) There are several possible donor groups on the DNA molecule that could bind magnesium ion in a specific way in addition to the possibly dominant phosphate residues. 2) The DNA molecules may be imperfect in that there can be nicks in the strands providing more than one type of phosphate residue; however, measurements of the nick concentrations indicate that this contribution should be small [23]. 3) By hypothesis we anticipate at least two types of magnesium-DNA interaction: domain binding that is weak and labile, and site binding that is relatively strong and less labile.

The nonlorentzian line shape apparent in Fig. 1b presents additional difficulties for analysis. Relaxation of a spin 5/2 nucleus will be non-exponential any time the extreme narrowing condition is violated. Clearly that must be the case for magnesium ion coordinated to a phosphate residue on DNA, but it is much less clear for a domain bound ion. The general treatment of the problem by Hubbard [24] has been extended by Bull and coworkers [25] specifically to the fast exchange case for spin 5/2 and 7/2 nuclei that sample nonextreme narrowing sites. For ^{25}Mg the treatment predicts three transverse relaxation rate constants that would result in a line shape that is similar to that shown in Fig. 1b. However, it does not appear that the analysis may be applied directly in the present system because the temperature dependence of the ^{25}Mg NMR line demonstrates that a significant fraction of the line shape falls into what may be loosely called a slow or intermediate exchange region with respect to the relaxation times at DNA sites [26]. In the case where magnesium ion exchange is slow, it is difficult to see that the distorted line shape should arise from the slow sampling of the DNA sites. An alternate possibility is that the solution is inhomogeneous in some way with respect to magnesium ion. Gels and ordered phases in DNA solutions are known, though none were readily apparent in the DNA solutions studied here [27]. It is important to note that the present DNA samples represent solutions of rigid rods and therefore there is a significant possibility that nonlorentzian behavior of the line could result from a partially developed quadrupole multiplet pattern. However the line shape is not significantly dependent on the DNA molecular weight nor is there clear evidence for a powder pattern under the central sharp line.

The general possibility of exchange limited relaxation rates raises an additional quantitative problem. The ^{25}Mg linewidth derived for magnesium bound to a monophosphate is of the order of 10^2 Hz. If we assume that there is at least a factor of a thousand change in correlation time on binding to a specific site on DNA, then the linewidth bound will be 10^5 Hz or larger. The fast exchange conditions thus require lifetimes for magnesium ions site-bound to DNA that are several orders of magnitude smaller than generally reported for simple phosphate systems. This estimate suggests that the contribution of site interactions to the magnesium NMR line may be kinetically attenuated by several orders of magnitude in this case and possibly in general. This conclusion adds an ambiguity to the present experiments in that a small number of magnesium ions that exchange rapidly with slow moving sites would make a disproportionate contribution to the linewidth. Thus, it is not possible at present to estimate the number of magnesium ions that are specifically bound in the present experiments and compare that with the total number of phosphate residues.

The two types of magnesium ion interaction with DNA or any polyelectrolyte, may be partly separated by taking advantage of ion competition experiments in which the magnesium ion is displaced from the site or the domain interactions preferentially. Sodium ion has very low affinity for phosphate oxygen sites and except for the indirect effects of total ionic strength, which is already high in these experiments, sodium ion should have minimal effect on the interaction between magnesium ions and phosphate groups on the DNA. On the other hand, sodium ion may compete favorably with the electrostatically entrapped divalent ions. Recognizing the possible difficulties with imcomplete line shape analysis, the full width measured at half maximum height of the ^{25}Mg line is plotted as a function of sodium concentration in Fig. 5. Several features of the data are important: 1) The titration curve demonstrates that the magnesium interaction with DNA is partially attenuated at high sodium ion concentration. 2) The linewidth plotted reaches a clear plateau at high sodium ion concentration. 3) The shape of the titration curve is reproducible but not described by a simple two site displacement model which is represented by the solid curve. 4) At the conclusion of the experiment the total ionic strength is high so that the distinction between a domain bound ion and the bulk solution may not be realistic and, in addition, the structure of the DNA may have changed. This last point provides a problem which may make clear distinctions between site binding and domain binding in polyelectrolytes difficult. At the low ionic strength limit where the ion condensation concepts work well, the concentrations may be such that specific site interactions are diluted away because of only moderate association constants.

The initial shape of the titration curve matches expectations for displacement of magnesium ion from the domain region in that the apparent displacement constant is 0.5. The deviations at higher concentrations may arise from failure of any of the assumptions used to calculate the titration

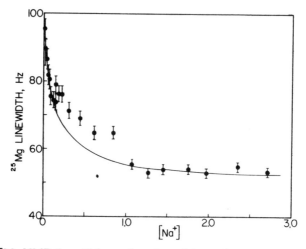

Figure 5. ^{25}Mg NMR linewidth as a function of the sodium ion concentration for a sample 77.2 mM in magnesium chloride and 14.8 mM in calf thymus DNA phosphate at 295 K. The solid curve represents the linewidth values expected if sodium ion displaces magnesium ion from the domain region with an equilibrium constant of 0.5.

curve: 1) The linewidth at half height for magnesium ion in the domain region is the same for all ions and independent of sodium ion concentration. 2) The ^{25}Mg line shape is constant as a function of sodium ion concentration. 3) All domain magnesium ions have the same apparent equilibrium constant for displacement by sodium ions. 4) No site interactions are involved in the displacement of magnesium observed. Measurements of the ^{25}Mg NMR linewidths at one quarter and three quarters height have shown that the line shape does change as a function of sodium concentration; hence, the linewidth at half height is not necessarily a simple or linear function of sodium concentration. We are unable to confirm the importance of the remaining factors that may lead to distortion of the titration curve at present.

   In spite of the several obvious interpretive complications, several conclusions are possible. While we have no reason to doubt the importance of nonspecific ion association with the DNA, and indeed, the sodium titration data in Fig. 5 could be used to support the hypothesis, it is also clear that site interactions make a substantial and probably dominant contribution to the magnesium NMR spectrum. A present frustration is that we are unable to show unambiguously that the spectrum is not dominated by a very few but very labile magnesium ion interactions. Hence quantitative assessment of the number of sites involved eludes us.

Acknowledgments

The authors gratefully acknowledge the support of this work by the following research grants: National Institutes of Health, GM-25757 (RGB) and National Science Foundation, PCM-7611016 (MTR).

References

1. A. White, R. Handler, and E. L. Smith, *Principles of Biochemistry*, McGraw-Hill, New York, 1968.
2. P. H. von Hippel and T. Schleich, *Acc. Chem. Res., 2*:257 (1969).
3. M. M. TaquiKhan and A. E. Martell, *J. Amer. Chem. Soc., 89*:5585 (1967).
4. M. Eigen in *Advances in the Chemistry of the Coordination Compounds*, (S. Kirschner, ed.), Macmillan, New York, 1961.
5. M. Eigen, *Pure and Applied Chemistry, 6*:97 (1963).
6. H. Diebler, M. Eigen, and G. G. Hammes, *Z. Naturforsch., 156*:554 (1969).
7. G. S. Manning, *Quart. Rev. Biophys., 11*:179 (1978).
8. C. F. Anderson, M. T. Record, Jr., and D. A. Hart, *Biophysical Chem., 7*:301 (1978).
9. J. A. Magnuson and A. A. Bothner-By in *Magnetic Resonance in Biological Research*, (A. Franconi, ed.), Gordon and Breach, London, 1969.
10. R. G. Bryant, *J. Mag. Reson., 6*:159 (1972).
11. P. Robertson, R. G. Hiskey, and K. A. Koehler, *J. Biol. Chem., 253*:5880 (1978).
12. P. Robertson, K. Koehler, and R. G. Hiskey, *Biochem. Biophys. Res. Comm., 86*:265 (1979).
13. A. Cave, J. Parello, T. Drakenberg, E. Thulin, and B. Lindman, *FEBS Lett., 100*:148 (1979).
14. E. O. Bishop, S. J. Kimber, B. E. Smith, and P. J. Beynon, *FEBS Lett., 101*:31 (1979).
15. P. Reimarsson, J. Parello, T. Drakenberg, H. Gustavson, and B. Lindman, *FEBS Lett., 108*:439 (1979).
16. F. H. Pollard and J. V. Martin, *Analyst, 81*:348 (1978).
17. A. Abragam, *Principles of Nuclear Magnetism*, The Clarendon Press, Oxford, 1961, Chapter 8.
18. H. P. Bennetto and E. F. Caldin, *J. Chem. Soc., A*, 2198 (1971).
19. L. Simeral and G. E. Maciel, *J. Chem. Phys., 80*:552 (1976).
20. T. J. Swift and R. E. Connick, *J. Chem. Phys., 37*:307 (1962).

21. P. Tovo, unpublished results.
22. M. L. Bleam, C. F. Anderson, and M. T. Record, Jr., submitted for publication (1980).
23. M. L. Bleam, C. F. Anderson, and M. T. Record, Jr., unpublished results.
24. P. S. Hubbard, *J. Chem. Phys., 53*:985 (1970).
25. T. E. Bull, S. Forsen, and D. L. Turner, *J. Chem. Phys., 70*:3106 (1979).
26. D. Murk Rose and R. G. Bryant, unpublished results.
27. V. A. Bloomfield, D. M. Crothers, and I. Tinoco, *Physical Chemistry of Nucleic Acids*, Harper and Row, New York, 1974.

CHAPTER 4

ELUCIDATION OF METALLOTHIONEIN STRUCTURE BY [113]Cd NMR

James D. Otvos* and Ian M. Armitage
The Department of Molecular Biophysics and Biochemistry
Yale University
New Haven, Connecticut

I. INTRODUCTION

Metallothioneins are a ubiquitous class of sulfhydryl-rich, low molecular weight proteins which are thought to play a central role in metal metabolism. Since the initial discovery in 1957 of the cadmium- and zinc-containing protein from equine kidney cortex [1], metallothioneins have been identified from a variety of other mammals (including man) and such widely divergent sources as birds, fish, microorganisms, and invertebrates [2,3]. The widespread occurrence of metallothionein in nature suggests that it serves an important biological function, though its exact role remains unclear. One hypothesis which has received by far the most attention is that the protein acts as a heavy metal detoxifying agent by sequestering cadmium, mercury, and perhaps other toxic metal ions. Bolstering this suggestion is the fact that exposure of many organisms to cadmium and mercury, as well as zinc and copper, causes rapid *de novo* synthesis of metallothionein which results in greatly elevated levels of the protein [4-7]. However, since zinc is found to be the major constituent of the protein isolated from animals which are not exposed to high levels of heavy metals [8,9], it is equally likely that metallothionein participates in normal zinc metabolism or homeostasis, perhaps serving in a storage or transport capacity. Other suggestions for the role of metallothionein have included

---

* Present affiliation: Department of Chemistry, University of Wisconsin, Milwaukee, Wisconsin

an involvement in copper metabolism, amino acid transport, and nucleic acid synthesis, transcription, or translation [8,10,11].

With a view towards reaching a better understanding of its function, we have been employing multinuclear NMR methods to define the structural details of the interactions which exist between metallothionein and its bound metal ions. Apart from extensive cysteine thiolate participation in metal ligation, little information has previously been available concerning the structure of the multiple metal binding sites and their spatial relationship with one another. This paucity of structural data exists primarily because of a failure as yet to obtain metallothionein crystals suitable for X-ray diffraction analysis and because of the "spectroscopically silent" nature of the metal ions most commonly bound to the protein. We have recently found that ^{113}Cd NMR provides a promising new method with which to probe the metal ion environments in the cadmium-containing protein [12]. In this chapter we will review the progress we have made to date using ^{113}Cd NMR in characterizing the structures of the metal binding sites in metallothionein from rabbit liver and crab (*Scylla serrata*) hepatopancreas.

A. Properties of Metallothionein

The metallothioneins which have been best characterized are those which are found in the cytosolic fraction of mammalian kidney and liver tissue. The distinguishing properties of the protein are its unusual amino acid composition and its high metal content. Of the 61 amino acid residues in the protein, 20 are cysteine residues [3] and each of them is known to participate in metal coordination via mercaptide linkages [13,14]. The other characteristic feature of its amino acid composition is the total absence of aromatic residues and histidine and the presence of relatively large amounts of serine and lysine. The maximum molar metal content of mammalian metallothioneins is reported to be 7 g-atoms per mole. However, many purified preparations of the protein contain somewhat less and often variable amounts of metal ion, presumably because loss of native metal can occur during the purification process. Little specific information exists regarding the structures of the 7 metal binding sites in metallothionein. Based on net charge considerations and the constant cysteine/metal ratio of about 3, it has been postulated that the metals exist as isolated, negatively charged trimercaptide complexes [15]. However, since mercaptide sulfur exhibits a pronounced tendency to bridge two or three adjacent metal ions [16], structures involving oligomeric metal binding sites are equally likely. Whether or not other protein residues besides cysteine participate in metal ligation is also unknown.

The identity of the metal ions bound to metallothionein is a function of the tissue origin of the protein as well as the history of exposure of the source animal to various metals. In animals not deliberately subjected to metal administration, zinc is found to be the main constituent of the liver protein while cadmium and zinc are present in roughly equal amounts in metallothionein from the kidney [8]. Following exposure of the animal to cadmium, zinc, copper, mercury, and other metals, not only does the isolated protein contain these metals, but the total metallothionein content in the tissues is found to be markedly increased. This induction process appears to occur at the transcriptional level [17,18], though the details of the triggering mechanism have yet to be worked out. Also not known is at what point in time the various metal ions become bound to the newly synthesized protein chains. In this regard it is interesting to note that in addition to the inducing metal, a significant amount of zinc is almost always found in the isolated protein. For example, even following administration of very high levels of cadmium, the induced metallothionein always contains about 30-40% zinc. Furthermore, the molar cadmium and zinc contents are usually nonintegral, indicating that the protein is heterogeneous with respect to metal composition. Of considerable interest is whether this heterogeneity arises from the presence of two populations of homogeneous metallothioneins, one containing zinc and the other cadmium, or whether there are several species present, each of which contains cadmium and zinc in different relative amounts. If the latter situation exists, one would like to know the distribution of zinc among the multiple binding sites in order to determine whether certain sites require zinc to maintain the structural integrity of the protein.

All metallothioneins which have been characterized to date can be separated by ion exchange chromatography into two major isoprotein forms designated MT-1 and MT-2. Sequence studies performed on the two isoproteins from several different sources indicate that the positions of the 20 cysteine residues as well as those of most of the serines and lysines are identical. The sequence differences which exist between MT-1 and MT-2 lie outside these highly conserved regions and are extensive enough to suggest that the isoproteins are coded by different cistrons. The two forms of the equine liver and kidney protein, for example, differ in 7 amino acid positions [19] while those from mouse liver differ in 15 positions [20]. It seems likely in view of the conservation of all 20 metal-coordinating cysteine residues and the presence in both isoproteins of 7 metal binding sites that the two forms of metallothionein perform identical functions. However, without a more detailed structural comparison between MT-1 and MT-2 it is impossible to rule out the existence of subtle functional differences between the two forms which might account for their evolutionary conservation.

B. Advantages of ^{113}Cd NMR as a Structural Probe

^{113}Cd NMR, which was first applied to the study of a biological system only four years ago [21], has subsequently been used to study a wide variety of metalloproteins in which the native Zn^{2+}, Cu^{2+}, Mg^{2+}, or Ca^{2+} ions are replaced by ^{113}Cd^{2+} [22-29]. The technique is particularly valuable because of its ability to provide a sensitive monitor of the metal ion environments in the many metalloproteins in nature which depend on the binding of diamagnetic, "spectroscopically-silent" metal ions for their functions. Although the catalytic activities of many of these enzymes are altered to some degree by the Cd^{2+} substitution, there is sufficient evidence regarding the coordination of Cd^{2+} in these systems to suggest that the structural and dynamic information derived from the ^{113}Cd NMR data provide an accurate representation of the native structures.

^{113}Cd is a particularly suitable metal nucleus for high resolution NMR studies of biological macromolecules because of its favorable magnetic properties. It has a spin quantum number $I = 1/2$ and relatively high sensitivity when observed at its natural abundance level of 12%. The eight-fold enhancement in sensitivity which is achieved by using the commercially-available ^{113}Cd isotope, enriched to >96 atom %, makes ^{113}Cd approximately 60 times more sensitive than ^{13}C at natural abundance. More importantly, ^{113}Cd also offers excellent spectral resolution resulting from the sensitivity of its chemical shift to very small differences in its coordination sphere. For the ^{113}Cd^{2+} - substituted metalloproteins examined to date, the range of observed chemical shifts exceeds 850 ppm! Noteworthy is the fact that in those cases where the protein ligands are known from other techniques, the ^{113}Cd chemical shifts follow the trends which were established several years ago for small inorganic complexes [30], where deshielding of the ^{113}Cd^{2+} ion was found to increase in the order $S > N > O$. For example, in parvalbumin where six oxygen atoms are ligated to the octahedrally-coordinated metal ions, the ^{113}Cd resonances appear at about - 100 ppm relative to 0.1M $Cd(ClO_4)_2$ [25]. At the other extreme, ^{113}Cd^{2+} substituted at the structural metal binding site of horse liver alcohol dehydrogenase, which contains four cysteine thiolate ligands arranged in a tetrahedral array, gives rise to the most deshielded ^{113}Cd resonance observed to date at 750 ppm [27].

The key to the study of metallothionein structure by ^{113}Cd NMR has turned out to be this remarkable sensitivity of ^{113}Cd^{2+} chemical shift to subtle differences in coordination environment. As we will show, it is possible to detect a resolved resonance from each of the seven metal ions in the protein, despite the fact that they all have very similar coordination sites. This has allowed us to characterize the extent and origin of the heterogeneity in the native Cd,Zn protein as well as the structural differences which exist between the two isoprotein forms. Since ^{113}Cd^{2+} is introduced into the metallothionein by inducing its synthesis *in vivo* with the enriched isotope, there can be no question that the ^{113}Cd NMR results pertain directly to the native structure of the protein.

II. CHARACTERIZATION OF RABBIT LIVER METALLOTHIONEIN

A. ^{113}Cd NMR Spectrum of Native Cd,Zn Metallothionein-2

The first ^{113}Cd NMR spectrum of metallothionein was taken at natural abundance using protein isolated from the livers of six rabbits which had been subjected to repeated injections of CdCl$_2$ [31]. The spectrum of this sample resulting from 39 hours of accumulation is shown in Figure 1A. Despite the very low signal to noise ratio, four resonances can be clearly identified within the chemical shift range of 614 to 668 ppm. By comparison with ^{113}Cd chemical shifts observed for a series of cadmium-alkylthiolate complexes [30] it could be inferred that the ^{113}Cd^{2+} ions giving rise to the four peaks must each be coordinated to at least three cysteine sulfur ligands and be located in sufficiently different chemical environments to allow their resolution by ^{113}Cd NMR.

Prompted by this encouraging result, the induction of the rabbit liver protein was repeated using isotopically-enriched 96 atom % ^{113}CdCl$_2$. The ^{113}Cd NMR spectrum of the MT-2 isoprotein isolated from these rabbit livers is shown in Figure 1B. As expected, a substantial improvement in signal to noise ratio is achieved by the use of the enriched isotope, allowing one to identify five resolved resonances appearing at 604, 613, 623, 641, and 668 ppm. As shown in Figure 1C, an improvement in spectral resolution can be obtained by employing proton decoupling to remove the unresolved proton couplings originating from the three-bond interaction of the ^{113}Cd^{2+} ions to the β protons of the multiple cysteine ligands. Under these conditions, it is now possible to resolve resonances from ^{113}Cd^{2+} located in at least six chemically distinct environments in the protein which is believed to contain seven metal binding sites.

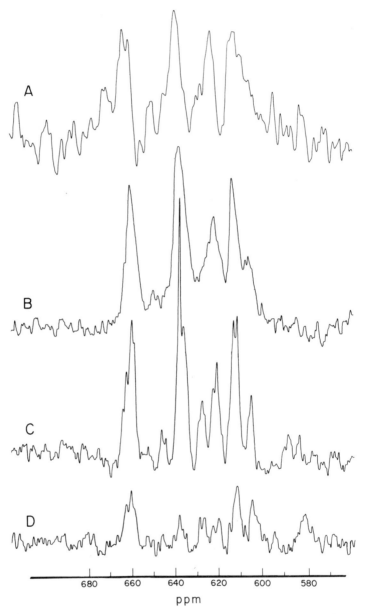

A

B

C

D

```
         680     660     640     620     600     580
                          ppm
```

Figure 1. [113]Cd NMR spectra at 19.96 MHz of rabbit liver Cd,Zn MT-2 (13mM) in 0.01M Tris, 0.1M NaCl, pH 8.8. A proton coupled spectrum (280,000 transients) of protein containing [113]Cd at natural abundance; B, proton coupled spectrum (7500 transients) of protein containing enriched (96 atom %) [113]Cd; C, gated proton decoupled spectrum (10,000 transients, 32 Hz digital broadening) of the same protein sample used in B; D, same as C but using continuous proton decoupling.

An important practical consideration in obtaining proton decoupled ^{113}Cd NMR spectra should be mentioned at this point. Because of the negative value of its magnetic moment, ^{113}Cd can experience nuclear Overhauser enhancements (NOE's), $\eta + 1$, which range from about +1 to -1.2 depending upon its correlation time [28]. For ^{113}Cd bound to metalloproteins, NOE values near zero are often observed, resulting in severe reductions or even loss of resonance intensity. Such an unfavorable situation exists for metallothionein. The proton decoupled spectrum shown in Figure 1C was acquired by gating the decoupler so that it is on only during acquisition, thereby eliminating the NOE. The spectrum in Figure 1D was obtained using the same spectral parameters, but with continuous proton decoupling to allow full development of the NOE. Clearly, the intensities of all of the resonances are reduced in Figure 1D, some to the extent that they are no longer observable. This result indicates that there is a large dipolar contribution to the overall relaxation of each ^{113}Cd^{2+} ion in metallothionein at this magnetic field strength and that significant, though as yet undefined, structural or dynamic differences exist in the multiple Cd^{2+} environments to account for the range of observed NOE values.

Upon closer examination of the gated proton decoupled spectrum in Figure 1C, replotted in Figure 2A using less digital broadening, one notices that each of the ^{113}Cd resonances contains considerable fine structure. The most attractive explanation for these splittings is that they arise from scalar coupling between adjacent ^{113}Cd^{2+} ions located in polynuclear clusters in the protein. An equally plausible, though perhaps less interesting, alternative is that the splittings represent small chemical shift differences which might arise from the metal ion heterogeneity of the native Cd,Zn metallothionein. Since the magnitudes of scalar couplings are field-independent, a simple method of distinguishing between these two alternatives is to acquire the ^{113}Cd spectrum at a different magnetic field strength. In Figure 2B is shown the ^{113}Cd NMR spectrum of the same sample of MT-2 taken at 2.2 times higher field strength. A careful comparison of the magnitude of the splittings in Figures 2A and B indicates that they indeed remain constant at the two fields, thereby establishing their origin as ^{113}Cd-^{113}Cd spin coupling. By analogy to known Cd^{2+}-thiolate polynuclear complexes [16,32-34], the spin couplings undoubtedly arise from a two-bond interaction between adjacent ^{113}Cd^{2+} ions mediated by one or more bridging cysteine sulfur ligands. The significance of this result is that it provides the first direct evidence that the metal ions in metallothionein exist in a polynuclear metal cluster arrangement rather than as isolated, trimercaptide complexes as had been generally assumed.

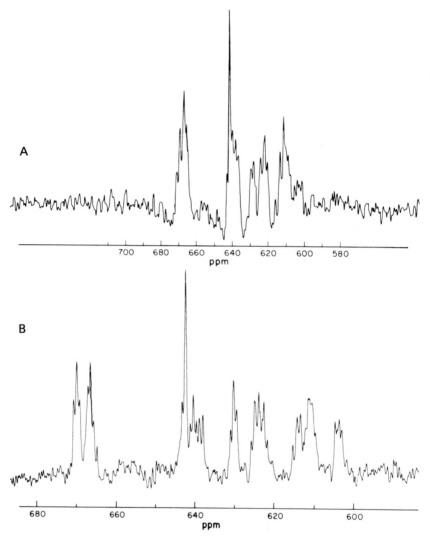

Figure 2. Proton decoupled ^{113}Cd NMR spectra of Cd,Zn MT-2 at two magnetic field strengths. A, 19.96 MHz spectrum (same spectrum as in Figure 1C) but treated with 11 Hz digital broadening; B, 44.4 MHz spectrum (4000 transients, 10 Hz digital broadening) plotted on the same frequency scale as A.

To our knowledge, metallothionein is the only system in which ^{113}Cd-^{113}Cd spin coupling has been observed. This is presumably a direct consequence of the stability of the metal-protein complex. Analogous couplings in similar ^{113}Cd^{2+}-alkylthiolate complexes in solution have not been observed [30,35], probably because of chemical exchange averaging resulting from ligand exchange processes which are fast compared with 1/J.

While most of the splittings in Figure 2A can be shown to arise from ^{113}Cd-^{113}Cd coupling, a few clearly result from chemical shift differences. The most easily visualized example of this is the downfield resonance at 668 ppm in Figure 2A, which at the higher field is separated into two peaks, each of which has residual splitting due to ^{113}Cd-^{113}Cd coupling (Figure 2B). With the increased resolution afforded by use of the higher field, it is apparent from the number of resonances observed in the spectrum in Figure 2B that ^{113}Cd^{2+} is located in more than seven chemically distinct environments despite the fact that metallothionein contains only seven metal binding sites. This observation confirms the suspected heterogeneity of the Cd,Zn protein which had previously been suggested as the origin of the nonintegral metal contents frequently found in native protein preparations. The metal composition of the MT-2 sample used to obtain the spectra in Figure 2, determined by atomic absorption and normalized to a total of 7 eq of metal/mole of protein, was 4.4 eq of Cd and 2.6 eq of Zn per mole. The ^{113}Cd NMR data clearly exclude the possibility that the heterogeneity which exists in this sample arises from the presence of only two homogeneous species, one containing Cd and the other Zn. If this were the case, one would expect to observe a maximum of only seven resolved ^{113}Cd multiplets. Since more than seven resonances are seen, the protein sample must consist of species which contain both Cd and Zn. A more detailed analysis of the spectrum is required before conclusions may be made concerning the number of protein species present and the extent to which Cd and Zn can substitute for one another at each of the seven binding sites in the protein.

B. Assignment of Multiplet Structure

1. Spin Echo Modulation

In order to extract additional structural information from the rather complex ^{113}Cd NMR spectrum of MT-2, it was first necessary to establish the exact number of resonances contained in the spectrum, the multiplet structure of each of them, and the connectivities between ^{113}Cd^{2+} ions in the protein which give rise to the different multiplets. As a first step towards achieving this goal, we employed a pulse method which has previously been shown to be helpful in interpreting complex ^{1}H NMR spectra of proteins [36]. The method is based on use of the normal spin echo pulse sequence $(90°\text{-}\tau\text{-}180°\text{-}\tau\text{-Acq})$ and takes advantage of the characteristic phase modulations which appear in the individual components of spin multiplets arising from homonuclear coupling [37]. The phase distortions, which evolve during the preparation period between the 90° pulse and the start of data acquisition $(T=2\tau)$ are directly related to the magnitude of the coupling constants and the nature of the spin multiplets. For example, while singlets exhibit no phase modulation, both components of a doublet are modulated at an angular frequency which causes them to be 180° out of phase with respect to the singlet when the total waiting period $T=1/J$. The central component of a triplet decays like a singlet, whereas the outer lines are modulated at twice the frequency of a doublet, so that at $T=1/2J$ they are inverted and at $T=1/J$ they are again back in phase with the central line.

The spectra in Figure 3 illustrate the value of this pulse method in assigning the multiplet structures of many of the resonances in the MT-2 spectrum. Each of the spin echo spectra was acquired under identical conditions (4 hours accumulation time each) with different values of the preparation period, T. Since the apparent coupling constants were measured to be about 30-50 Hz, the T values employed span a range up to about 1/J. The anticipated phase modulations resulting from the existence of extensive [113]Cd-[113]Cd spin coupling can be readily observed in most of the resonances in these spectra. Interestingly, the intense peak at 642 ppm was the only resonance in the spectrum which exhibited the behavior expected for a singlet (i.e., no phase change). The multiplicities of most of the other resonances were assigned relatively easily by analyzing the phase information contained in the spectra in Figure 3 and in similar spin echo spectra. An expansion of the spectrum taken with $T=12$ msec (about 1/2J for the couplings observed) is shown in Figure 4 in order to more clearly illustrate the nature of the observed phase modulations. At $T=1/2J$ the outer lines of any triplets* in the spectrum should be inverted with respect to the central line. This behavior is clearly seen in Figure 4 for the resonances at 670, 640, and 630 ppm. In contrast, the resonance centered at 667 ppm, which appears to be a triplet in the unmodulated $T=2$ msec

---

*Strictly speaking, the spectrum contains no triplets, but rather doublets of doublets since all of the [113]Cd^{2+} ions in the protein are chemically inequivalent. For convenience, however, we will routinely refer to the splittings arising from AXY and AXYZ systems as triplets and quartets, respectively.

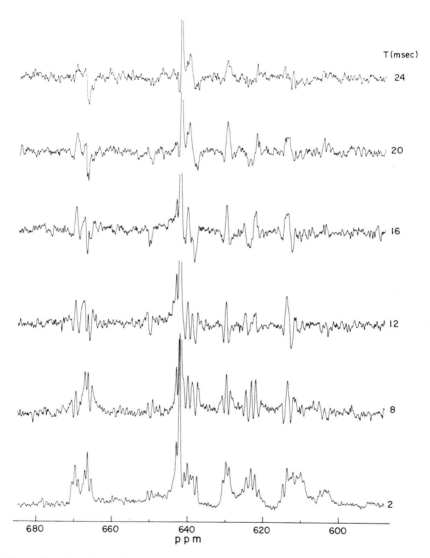

Figure 3. A series of spin echo spectra of Cd,Zn MT-2 at 44.4 MHz. Each spectrum was acquired using the indicated value of T, the time interval between the 90° pulse and the start of data acquisition.

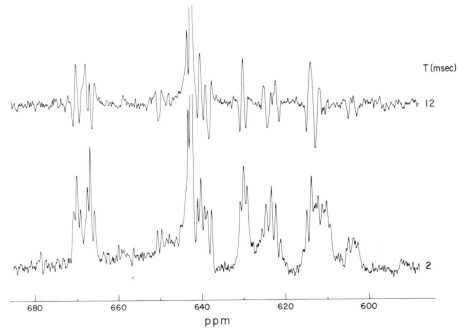

Figure 4.   An expanded view of the phase distortions in the Cd, Zn MT-2 spin echo spectrum (10,000 transients) when T = 12 msec.

spectrum, does not exhibit the expected phase change when T=2 msec. Additional spectra taken with T≈ 1/J show that this "triplet" is actually two overlapping doublets.

Despite its demonstrated usefulness, the application of the spin echo technique to metallothionein [113]Cd spectra suffers from several limitations. The main limitation arises from the amount of T_2 relaxation which occurs during the waiting period 2τ, resulting in severely diminished signal intensities when the waiting period exceeds 1/2J. The progressive reduction in signal to noise which accompanies increasing delay times can be clearly seen in Figure 3. Differences in the T_2 values of individual resonances in the spectrum are also apparent from the differential rates at which they disappear with increasing values of T. Another problem which complicates the assignment of overlapping resonances is the fact that the coupling constants are not all identical, but instead vary from 30-50 Hz. Thus, it is impossible using a single delay time to generate phase angles which are the same for all doublets, triplets, and quartets in the spectrum. Many assignments are therefore difficult to make simply by visual inspection of the data. However, by transforming the spin echo spectra into a 2-

dimensional J-resolved data set [38] the assignment problem can be greatly simplified. 2D ^{113}Cd NMR spectra of metallothionein have, in fact, been acquired [35] and an example is shown later (see Section IV, Figure 15).

2. Long-Range Coupling

In addition to 2-bond coupling (30-50 Hz) arising from interactions between adjacent ^{113}Cd^{2+} ions linked by bridging thiolate ligands, a close inspection of the MT-2 spectrum also reveals smaller couplings of 5-7 Hz in four of the ^{113}Cd resonances. These small couplings, whose identification helped elucidate the final structures of the MT-2 clusters, result from a 4-bond interaction between ^{113}Cd^{2+} ions which are next nearest neighbors in the same cluster. As shown in the expanded view of the downfield half of the MT-2 spectrum in Figure 5, the long-range couplings in three of the resonances are clearly distinguishable: the outer lines of the triplet at 670 ppm are split into doublets, the doublet at 666 ppm is split (while the overlapping doublet at 668 ppm is not), and the doublet at 638 ppm is also

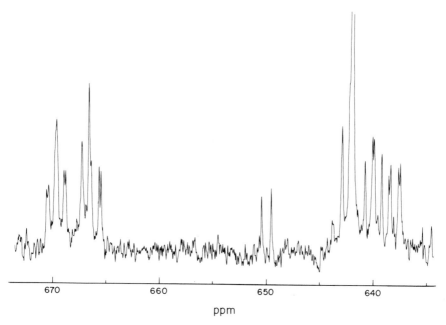

Figure 5. The downfield half of a proton decoupled ^{113}Cd NMR spectrum of Cd,Zn MT-2 treated with 3 Hz digital broadening.

split. Though not shown in Figure 5, the triplet at 630 ppm is also involved in a long-range interaction with a single $^{113}Cd^{2+}$ ion.

3. Homonuclear Decoupling

By performing a series of homonuclear decoupling experiments, in which each ^{113}Cd multiplet in the spectrum was subjected in turn to a selective decoupling pulse, it was possible to establish the linkages which exist between every $^{113}Cd^{2+}$ ion in the protein. With this information, definite conclusions could be made regarding the number of metal clusters in metallothionein, their size and structure, and the extent and origin of the heterogeneity which is introduced into the native protein by the presence of Zn.

In Figures 6A and B are shown two examples of homonuclear decoupled MT-2 spectra. The frequencies at which the decoupling pulses were applied are indicated by the arrows and each collapsed or partially collapsed multiplet is identified by an 'X'. Analysis of these and similar spectra was quite straightforward. In Figure 6A, for example, the relatively strong decoupling pulse applied at the center of the complex multiplet at 623 ppm resulted in collapse of the triplet at 670 ppm to a doublet, collapse of one of the two overlapping doublets at 666 ppm to a singlet, and so forth.

A summation of the information provided by both the spin echo modulation and homonuclear decoupling experiments is presented in Figure 7. The ^{113}Cd spectrum of MT-2 was shown to contain 15 separate resonances, whose multiplicities are indicated beneath the spectrum. The connections between the coupled multiplets are shown above the spectrum. The homonuclear decoupling results indicate that the 15 ^{113}Cd resonances arise from Cd^{2+} located in only 6 discrete assemblages of metal ion: one set contains 4 Cd^{2+} ions, two sets contain 3 Cd^{2+} ions, two sets contain 2 Cd^{2+} ions, and the sixth set contains only a single Cd^{2+} ion. From this information alone, it is obvious that the heterogeneity introduced by the presence of Zn in native MT-2 is quite limited. If Cd and Zn were randomly distributed among the 7 binding sites in the protein, we would have expected to observe a much more complex spectrum containing many additional sets of ^{113}Cd resonances.

Despite the limited extent of metal ion heterogeneity, the ^{113}Cd NMR spectrum of native MT-2 does not unfortunately lend itself to unambiguous interpretation with regard to the size and structure of its metal clusters. The problem is simply the uncertainty which exists regarding the exact locations of the Zn^{2+} ions. For example, the fact that the largest

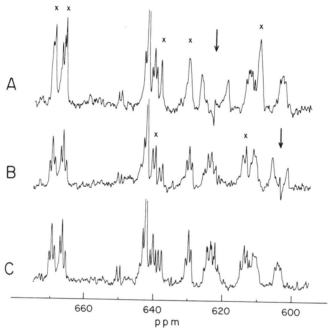

Figure 6. The effects of [113]Cd homonuclear decoupling on the Cd,Zn MT-2 spectrum. A normal proton decoupled spectrum (7200 transients, 8 Hz digital broadening) is shown in trace C. Spectra A and B were acquired under identical conditions with selective homonuclear decoupling pulses applied at the frequencies indicated by the arrows. Each of the collapsed multiplets is identified by an 'X'.

metal cluster identified by the NMR data contains 4 Cd^{2+} ions does not necessarily indicate that this is the size of one of the clusters in the protein. Without additional information the possibility cannot be ruled out that a 5-, 6-, or 7-metal cluster is actually present which always contains Zn^{2+} at certain of the binding sites.

An obvious solution to this problem would be to replace all the Zn^{2+} ions in the native protein with $^{113}Cd^{2+}$, thereby generating a homogeneous sample whose [113]Cd NMR spectrum should be considerably simpler as well as lending itself to unambiguous interpretation. In the next section we will outline the results of such a study on homogeneous [113]Cd metallothionein. Using the structural information obtained from this data, we will then return in Section IID to discuss the probable metal ion composition of the clusters in native Cd,Zn MT-2.

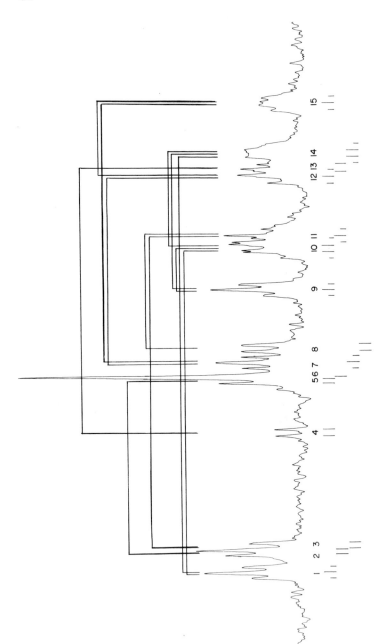

Figure 7. A "fully-relaxed" proton decoupled 113Cd spectrum at 44.4 MHz of Cd,Zn MT-2. The spectrum (2700 transients) was acquired using a 90° pulse, 8 second recycle time, and gated proton decoupling. Beneath the spectrum are indicated the multiplet structures of each of the 15 resonances. Above are shown the 2-bond spin coupling connections between the individual resonances as determined by the homonuclear decoupling data.

C. Metal Cluster Structure of Homogeneous Cd Metallothionein

Since metallothioneins from mammalian sources always contain Zn, no matter how much Cd is administered to the animal, it is necessary to exchange the native Zn for Cd in vitro to obtain the homogeneous Cd protein. We find that by adding excess ^{113}Cd^{2+} to the liver homogenate prior to performing the initial gel filtration step in the purification procedure it is possible to displace virtually all of the Zn^{2+} with ^{113}Cd^{2+} [39].

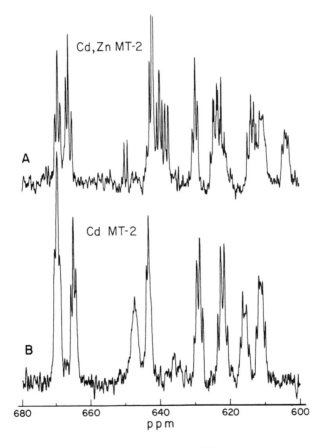

Figure 8. Comparison of the proton decoupled ^{113}Cd NMR spectra of native Cd,Zn MT-2 (A) and homogeneous Cd MT-2 (B), prepared by replacing the native Zn in vitro as described in the text.

Cysteine oxidation is kept to a minimum using this procedure, unlike dialysis of the purified protein against Cd^{2+} which is usually accompanied by significant disulfide formation [35].

The ^{113}Cd NMR spectrum of homogeneous Cd MT-2 (Cd:Zn = 45:1) is compared to the spectrum of the native Cd,Zn protein (Cd:Zn = 1.8:1) in Figure 8. As expected, the spectrum of the Cd protein is considerably less complex than that of the native protein, containing only 8 resonances instead of 15. It is noteworthy that while several resonances in the two spectra have identical chemical shifts, the three multiplets at 648, 644, and 616 ppm in the Cd MT-2 spectrum have no counterparts in the Cd,Zn MT-2 spectrum. Assuming that a "native" structure is generated by our *in vitro* metal exchange procedure, this result provides evidence that none of the species which comprise the heterogeneous native Cd,Zn MT-2 sample is a homogeneous seven-Cd metallothionein.

For some period of time we were quite puzzled by the presence of 8 ^{113}Cd resonances in the spectrum of the homogeneous Cd protein since metallothionein is known to bind only 7 metal ions. Also puzzling were the results of several homonuclear decoupling experiments which were performed to help unravel the structure of the protein's polynuclear metal cluster(s). In many cases it was observed that resonances which were affected by a particular homonuclear decoupling pulse did not collapse into readily identifiable multiplets. The reason for this behavior became clear once it was realized that the Cd-MT-2 spectrum is actually more complex than it appears.

The key experiment which provided the insight needed to interpret the NMR data was to simply acquire a "fully relaxed" spectrum (pulse repetition rate > $4T_1$ gated ^1H decoupling) as shown in Figure 9*. Under these conditions, where the resonance amplitudes are a direct measure of the concentrations of the individual $^{113}Cd^{2+}$ ions in the protein, it is clear that the two multiplets labeled 7 and 7' each represent about half the amount of $^{113}Cd^{2+}$ as do the three resonances at 670, 630, and 622 ppm. This fact, in conjunction with homonuclear decoupling results which showed that all of these resonances are connected with one another, allowed us to conclude that metallothionein contains a 4-metal cluster which we have designated

---

*The MT-1 isoprotein was used to obtain the spectrum in Figure 9 because it was available in larger amounts than MT-2. As will be discussed in Section III, the two isoproteins exhibit identical ^{113}Cd NMR spectra (and hence have identical metal cluster structures) and may therefore be used interchangeably.

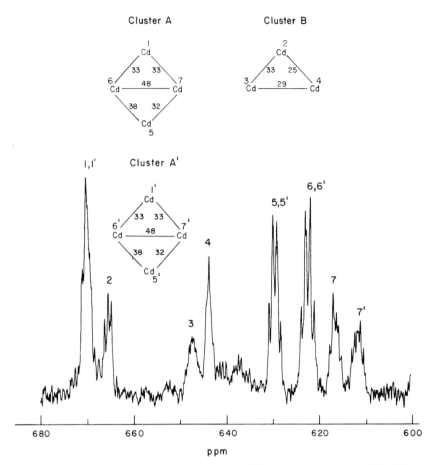

Figure 9. A "fully relaxed" proton decoupled ^{113}Cd NMR spectrum of Cd MT-1 and schematic representations of the metal cluster structures in the protein, established by homonuclear decoupling experiments (see text). The spectrum was acquired using a 90° pulse, 8 second recycle time, and gated proton decoupling. The spin coupling connections which were shown to exist between adjacent metal ions in the clusters are indicated by the lines connecting the Cd ions in the schematic structures. The number beside each Cd refers to its corresponding resonance in the ^{113}Cd spectrum and the numbers appearing on the lines connecting the metals are the measured 2-bond coupling constants ($\pm$ 3 Hz). The cysteine thiolate ligands which bridge the adjacent metals have been omitted from the drawings for clarity.

as cluster A. The confusing NMR properties of the Cd protein sample stem from the fact that cluster A apparently exists in two forms, A and A', which are present in approximately equal concentrations. Because the two forms differ in an as yet undefined way in structure or conformation, or the environment of the cluster is different in two classes of protein species, the resonances corresponding to the $^{113}Cd^{2+}$ ions at the 4 binding sites in the cluster exhibit different chemical shifts. One of the 4 Cd^{2+} ions is particularly sensitive to the difference between the two forms, giving rise to resonance 7 in cluster A and resonance 7' in cluster A'. The Cd^{2+} ions at the other 3 sites in the cluster are much less affected, giving rise to overlapping multiplets centered at 670, 630, and 622 ppm which differ in chemical shift by only 15, 45, and 5 Hz, respectively. The two forms of cluster A are represented diagrammatically in Figure 9. The observed 2-bond coupling constants are indicated next to the lines connecting the Cd^{2+} ions and the bridging thiolate ligands have been omitted for clarity.

As demonstrated by additional homonuclear decoupling experiments, the remaining Cd^{2+} ions in metallothionein are located in a 3-metal cluster, cluster B, whose structure is also depicted in Figure 9. It is interesting to note that the resonances corresponding to the 3 metal ions in cluster B, resonances 2, 3, and 4, have significantly smaller integrated areas than the resonances arising from the $^{113}Cd^{2+}$ ions located in cluster A, all of which have very nearly equal areas. In addition, the multiplet structures of peaks 2, 3, and 4 are somewhat less well defined than those of the other resonances. We interpret these observations as indicating that cluster B is partially deficient in $^{113}Cd^{2+}$, either because of nonspecific loss of $^{113}Cd^{2+}$ from these sites during protein purification and storage or because the original Cd,Zn protein in the liver homogenate had already irreversibly lost some cluster B metal ion prior to the exahange of Zn^{2+} with $^{113}Cd^{2+}$. Similar observations on metallothionein samples from other preparations lead us to believe that the metals in cluster B are indeed more labile than those in cluster A. Metal exchange experiments are currently underway to quantitate the extent of this differential lability.

Having established that the seven metal ions in rabbit liver metallo-thionein are arranged in such a way as to form the two metal clusters shown schematically in Figure 9, it was of considerable interest to determine whether structures consistent with the NMR data could be drawn which would also account for the known involvement of all 20 cysteine residues in metal ligation. In Figure 10 are shown postulated structures of cluster A and cluster B which satisfy all of the spin coupling information provided by the ^{113}Cd NMR data. All metal ions are depicted as being

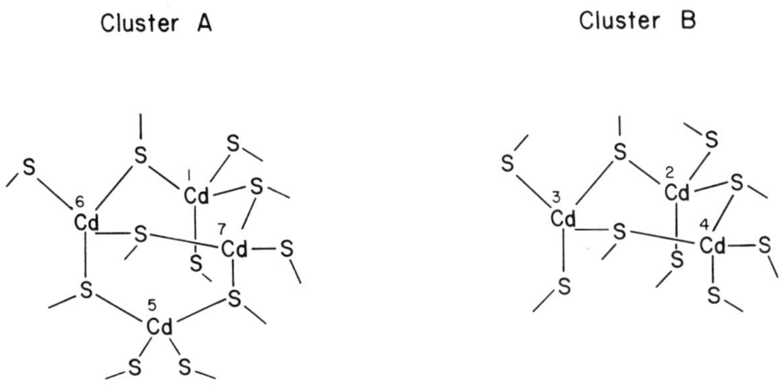

Cluster A   Cluster B

Figure 10. Postulated structures of the 4-metal and 3-metal clusters in rabbit liver metallothionein based on the spin coupling information contained in the Cd MT-1 spectrum and on considerations discussed in the text.

tetrahedrally coordinated to 4 thiolate ligands on the basis of [113]Cd chemical shift considerations [27,30] and optical studies on Co^{2+}-substituted metallothionein [40]. Satisfyingly, these two structures turn out to require all 20 of the cysteine residues in the protein, eleven in cluster A and nine in cluster B. All adjacent metal ions are linked to one another by single bridging thiolate ligands, unlike some model Cd-thiolate complexes which utilize two bridging sulfur atoms [16]. As depicted in Figure 10, the 7 Cd^{2+} ions in the protein are situated in two types of sites. Two metals (labeled 6 and 7) are coordinated by 3 bridging sulfur ligands and one nonbridging sulfur and these give rise to the most shielded resonances in the spectrum. The other five metals are each liganded to 2 bridging and 2 nonbridging thiolates and give rise to more deshielded resonances. Although the coordination spheres of each of the two types of metal ions are depicted as being identical in Figure 10, sufficient differences must exist in the surrounding protein structure of each metal ion to induce the [113]Cd chemical shift and spin coupling differences which are observed.

D. Metal Cluster Structure of Native Cd,Zn Metallothionein-2

With the structural information provided by the preceeding analysis of the [113]Cd NMR properties of Cd metallothionein, we may now return to the data presented in Figure 7 and draw some conclusions regarding the metal cluster composition of the heterogeneous Cd,Zn protein. As was discussed in Section IIB, the 15 ^{113}Cd resonances in the Cd,Zn MT-2 spectrum in Figure 7 were assigned on the basis of homonuclear decoupling experiments as arising from ^{113}Cd^{2+} ions linked to one another in 6 discrete clusters. In Figure 11 are shown schematic structures of these 6 groups of ^{113}Cd^{2+} ions based on the chemical shift and spin coupling information contained in Figure 7 and on the assumptions discussed below. The number beside each Cd refers to the corresponding resonance in the spectrum in Figure 7 and the measured 2-bond coupling constants are indicated on the lines connecting the metals. In parentheses are indicated the relative amounts of each of the 6 Cd-containing clusters in the sample as determined by integration of a "fully relaxed" spectrum.

Only one of the 6 clusters in the native protein, the one containing the 4 ^{113}Cd^{2+} ions which give rise to resonances 1, 9, 10, and 14, can be unambiguously identified as a type A cluster. The chemical shifts and spin coupling parameters of the 4 resonances are identical within experimental error to those which were previously assigned to cluster A' in the Cd MT spectrum in Figure 9. Unfortunately, none of the other clusters in Cd,Zn MT-2 may be similarly assigned as type B clusters since there are no resonances in Figure 7 located at the chemical shift positions occupied by the cluster B resonances 3 and 4 in Figure 9. For this reason, certain assumptions need to be made in order to categorize the remaining 5 clusters as shown in Figure 11. The main assumption is that the ^{113}Cd chemical shifts in metallothionein are determined primarily by the structural characteristics of the 7 individual binding sites in the molecule (i.e., by the identity and geometrical arrangement of the protein ligands to the metal at the different sites and by their spacial locations within the surrounding protein structure). The actual metal ion compositions of the clusters are assumed to be less important determinants of chemical shift. Therefore, relatively small chemical shift differences are anticipated for ^{113}Cd^{2+} located at a particular cluster site in protein species which differ from one another only by the substitution of Zn^{2+} for Cd^{2+} at one or more of the other binding sites in the same cluster. Based on this assumption and the results of the previous section, which indicated that all of the relatively shielded resonances located upfield of 625 ppm correspond to Cd^{2+} ions in cluster A which are linked by bridging thiolate ligands to 3 adjacent metal ions, we can reasonably expect that the resonances in the upfield region of the Cd,Zn MT-2 spectrum also arise from Cd^{2+} ions located in these positions of type A clusters. On this basis, resonances 10-15 in Figure 7 were assigned to Cd^{2+} ions occupying such sites, which in turn identified 4 of the 6 Cd-containing clusters in the heterogeneous MT-

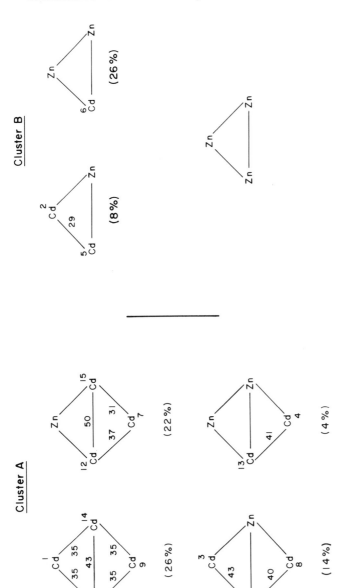

Figure 11. Proposed structures of the metal clusters which give rise to the 6 sets of ^{113}Cd resonances in the native Cd,Zn MT-2 spectrum. The number beside each Cd refers to the corresponding resonances in the native MT-2 spectrum in Figure 7. The observed 2-bond coupling constants ($\pm$ 3 Hz) are indicated on the lines connecting adjacent Cd ions. Bridging thiolate ligands have been omitted from the structures for clarity. In parentheses are given the relative amounts of each Cd-containing cluster in the native protein as determined by integration of the spectrum in Figure 7.

2 sample as type A clusters. In the postulated structures of these clusters shown in Figure 11, the locations of the Zn and Cd were assigned in such a way as to conform to all of the homonuclear decoupling results and to give the closest possible chemical shift correspondence between Cd^{2+} ions in different species bound to the same cluster position. The same considerations were used in proposing the structure of the 2 type B clusters.

The most interesting conclusion which emerges from the above analysis is that the overwhelming majority of the Cd^{2+} in the native Cd,Zn protein is located in type A clusters. Integration of the MT-2 spectrum indicates that 84% of the total ^{113}Cd resonance intensity is attributable to $^{113}Cd^{2+}$ bound to 4-metal clusters. Based on the postulated structures in Figure 11, 2 of the 4 sites in cluster A are apparently always occupied by Cd^{2+}, whereas the remaining 2 sites are susceptible to Zn^{2+} substitution. Most of the Zn^{2+} in native MT-2, on the other hand, is located in type B clusters. Cd^{2+} can be found to occupy 2 of the 3 binding sites in cluster B, but the third appears to always contain Zn^{2+}. Indirect evidence also indicates that a sizeable fraction of the native Cd,Zn protein consists of species which contain type B clusters occupied only by Zn^{2+}, which makes them undetectable by ^{113}Cd NMR. The existence of these "invisible" Zn^{2+} clusters is required to account for the known Zn^{2+} content of the protein sample and to explain the imbalance which is observed in the relative amounts of type A and type B clusters determined by integration of the MT-2 spectrum.

III. COMPARISON OF RABBIT LIVER METALLOTHIONEIN ISOPROTEINS

Current evidence indicates that the two major isoproteins of metallothionein, MT-1 and MT-2, have been conserved throughout the evolution of vertebrates and invertebrates [41]. The amino acid differences which exist between the two isoproteins have all been found to occur outside the highly conserved region of the sequences occupied by all 20 of the metal-coordinating cysteine residues [3]. For this reason, it has been assumed that MT-1 and MT-2 interact in an identical manner with their bound metal ions and also perform identical biological functions. However, since no direct evidence exists to substantiate these ideas, it was of interest to compare the structures of rabbit liver MT-1 and MT-2 using ^{113}Cd NMR.

In Figure 12 are shown spectra of the two homogeneous ^{113}Cd isoproteins. Remarkably, the two spectra are virtually identical, indicating that when Cd^{2+} is allowed to occupy all seven of the binding sites in the

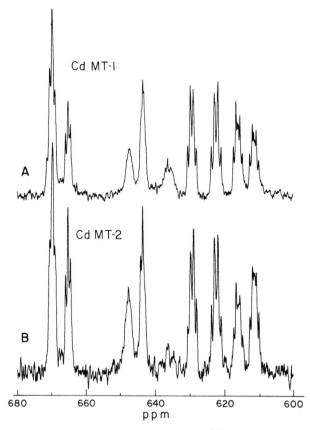

Figure 12. Comparison of the proton decoupled [113]Cd NMR spectra of homogeneous Cd MT-1 (A) and Cd MT-2 (B).

protein, MT-1 and MT-2 adopt identical metal cluster structures. The situation is quite different, however, for the native Cd,Zn isoproteins, as shown by their [113]Cd NMR spectra in Figure 13. While the two spectra are in many respects very similar, significant differences are observed which most likely reflect a different distribution of Zn^{2+} and Cd^{2+} among the multiple binding sites in the two isoproteins and perhaps also subtle structural differences in the metal clusters themselves. Particularly interesting is the observation that only one of the two forms of type A cluster (cluster A') is present in native MT-2 while both forms exist in MT-1. This fact is indicated most clearly by the presence and absence in MT-1 and MT-2, respectively, of the overlapping resonances at 670 and 630 ppm which

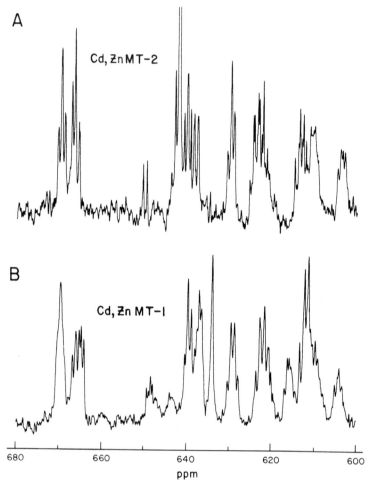

Figure 13. Comparison of the proton decoupled ^{113}Cd NMR spectra of native Cd,Zn MT-2 (A) and Cd,Zn MT-1 (B).

were attributed in Section IIC to the coexistence of the two forms of type A cluster. Whatever the origin may be of this difference and the others which exist between the two isoproteins, it is important to note that different preparations of native MT-1 and MT-2 always exhibit identical ^{113}Cd NMR spectra. Thus, it would appear that the number, metal composition, and relative amounts of the cluster species which are present in the heterogeneous Cd,Zn protein are not only quite different for the two isoproteins but are completely reproducible as well. In view of this finding, it is not inconceivable that functional differences indeed may exist between MT-1 and MT-2.

IV. CHARACTERIZATION OF AN INVERTEBRATE METALLOTHIONEIN

In collaboration with Dr. R. W. Olafson, we have recently begun an investigation of a crustacean metallothionein isolated from mud crab (*Scylla serrata*) hepatopancreas. Despite the evolutionary distance between crustaceans and mammals, the crab metallothionein exhibits many physical properties which are very similar to those of mammalian metallothioneins [41]. The protein can be induced by the administration of cadmium [42] and exists in two major isoprotein forms [41]. According to the recently completed sequence, crab MT-1 contains 58 amino acid residues, 18 of which are cysteine residues [43]. Only about 59% sequence homology exists between the crab and mammalian metallothioneins, reflecting their distant evolutionary relatedness. In view of this fact, we were interested in determining by ^{113}Cd NMR whether the metal ions bound to the crab protein are arranged in polynuclear clusters and, if so, how their structures compare with those found in the rabbit liver protein.

Fortuitously, crab MT-1 is particularly amenable to ^{113}Cd NMR investigation since the protein isolated from ^{113}Cd $^{2+}$-injected crabs contains virtually no Zn^{2+} [41]. The native ^{113}Cd protein is therefore homogeneous and consequently exhibits an uncomplicated NMR spectrum, as shown in Figure 14A. Five resolved multiplets are detected between 620 and 660 ppm. Integration of a "fully relaxed" spectrum indicates that the resonances labeled 1, 2, 5, and 6 each arise from single ^{113}Cd^{2+} ions while the multiplet at 647 ppm represents 2 ^{113}Cd^{2+} ions. Since each resonance in the spectrum exhibits ^{113}Cd-^{113}Cd spin coupling, it is apparent that all 6 ^{113}Cd^{2+} ions in the protein are indeed located in polynuclear metal clusters. Determination of the structure of these clusters was achieved by performing selective homonuclear decoupling experiments, two of which are shown in Figures 14B and C. The spectrum in Figure 14B demonstrates that decoupling resonance 1 causes the collapse of resonances 2 and 6 into doublets, while application of the decoupling pulse to the overlapping resonances 3 and 4 in Figure 14C causes the collapse of resonance 5 from a triplet to a singlet. From these two experiments alone, it may be concluded that the metals in crab MT-1 are situated in two 3-metal clusters, one containing the ^{113}Cd^{2+} ions giving rise to resonances 1, 2, and 6 and the other containing the metals corresponding

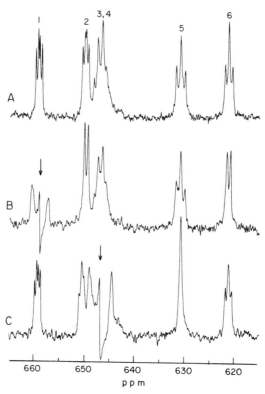

Figure 14. ^{113}Cd NMR spectra at 44.4 MHz of native crab MT-1 (8mM; Cd:Zn=60:1) in 0.01M Tris, 0.1M NaCl, pH 9.0. A proton decoupled spectrum (23,000 transients; 3 Hz digital broadening); B and C, same as A but with homonuclear decoupling pulses applied at the frequencies indicated by the arrows.

to resonances 3, 4, and 5. Both clusters are arranged such that each metal is linked to the two adjacent metals in the cluster. These structures therefore appear to be identical to the type B clusters found in rabbit liver metallothionein. Consistent with this idea is the fact that crab MT-1 contains 18 cysteine residues, exactly the number required to form two type B clusters having the structure proposed in Figure 10. It is quite interesting that despite a lack of extensive sequence homology between the crab and mammalian metallothioneins, both proteins appear to interact with metal in very similar manners. This suggests that whatever the physiological role(s) of metallothionein may be, its function is in some way related to its ability to form well-defined metal cluster structures of the type depicted in Figure 10.

More for academic interest than to provide additional structural information, we have recently used the crab protein to assess the practicality of using two-dimensional J-resolved spectroscopy as a routine method of interpreting the complex [113]Cd-[113]Cd spin coupling patterns which are often found in [113]Cd metallothionein spectra. The main advantage of the technique, which spreads out a weakly homonuclear coupled spectrum into chemical shift and spin coupling dimensions [38], is that in a single experiment the multiplet structures of severely overlapping resonances can be easily assigned. However, a serious drawback in terms of application to protein systems and nuclei other than protons is the amount of time required to accumulate the multiple spin echo spectra which make up the 2D data set. In Figure 15 is shown a two-dimensional [113]Cd NMR spectrum of crab MT-1 (8 mM in 2 ml) which was acquired in 60 hours.

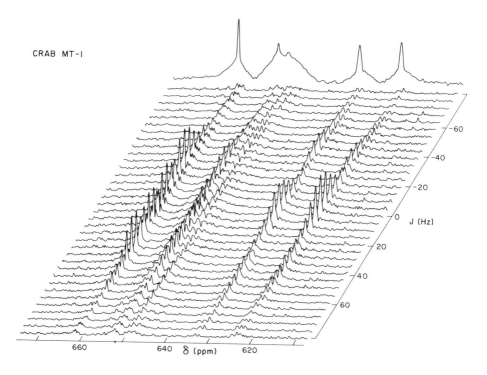

Figure 15. Two-dimensional J-resolved [113]Cd NMR spectra of crab MT-1 computed from 2D individual spin echo spectra (3 hours each). The top trace is the fully [113]Cd decoupled spectrum obtained by projecting the 2D spectrum onto the chemical shift (δ) axis.

The completely homonuclear decoupled ^{113}Cd spectrum obtained by projecting the 2D spectrum onto the chemical shift axis is shown in the uppermost trace. The good signal to noise characteristics of this spectrum clearly indicate that the application of 2D J-resolved spectroscopy to the metallothionein system is not only feasible but should find extensive application in future studies, particularly on heterogeneous protein samples.

V. CONCLUSIONS

For several reasons, few of which were anticipated when the studies were initiated, ^{113}Cd NMR has proven to be an exceptionally rich source of structural information on metallothionein. The key finding was the observation of well-resolved ^{113}Cd-^{113}Cd spin coupling in each of the resonances appearing in the ^{1}H-decoupled spectra. Not only did this prove that the metal ions in metallothionein are linked to one another by bridging cysteine thiolate ligands to form polynuclear clusters, but it allowed their structures to be determined by the combined use of spin echo modulation and homonuclear decoupling techniques. It was shown that rabbit liver metallothionein contains two separate metal clusters, one containing 4 metals and the other 3. These structures are almost certainly shared by all mammalian metallothionein judging by the extensive homologies which exist in their amino acid sequences. A distantly-related crustacean metallothionein was also demonstrated to contain two separate metal clusters (3 metals in each) which suggests that the two-cluster arrangement of the metal ions in metallothionein is conserved throughout evolution, presumably because such an arrangement is linked to its biological function (as yet unknown). Determination of the extent and origin of the heterogeneity which exists in native Cd,Zn metallothionein has also been possible using ^{113}Cd NMR, owing to the sensitivity of the ^{113}Cd chemical shifts to the presence of Zn^{2+} at neighboring sites in the clusters. It was found that about 85% of the Cd in Cd,Zn MT-2 is bound to the 4-metal cluster while most of the Zn is located in the 3-metal cluster. The distribution of Cd and Zn among the multiple binding sites is different for native MT-1 and MT-2, but for each isoprotein is completely reproducible. Interestingly, the two isoproteins do not appear to differ with regard to the cluster structures which are formed when Cd is the only metal ion bound to the protein.

Acknowledgments

We thank Dr. R. W. Olafson for his generous gift of the crab metallothionein and Carla Forte for her excellent technical assistance in isolating the rabbit liver protein. Funding for this work was provided by NIH Grant ES 01674 from the National Institute of Environmental Health Services, NIH Grant AM 18778, and NSF Grant PCM77-18941.

References

1. M. Margoshes and B. L. Vallee, *J. Amer. Chem. Soc., 79*: 4813 (1957).
2. Y. Kojima and J. H. R. Kagi, *Trends Biochem. Sci.*: 90 (1978).
3. M. Nordberg and Y. Kojima, "Report from the First International Meeting on Metallothionein and other Low Molecular Weight Metal-Binding Proteins" in *Metallothionein* (J. H. R. Kägi and M. Nordberg, eds.), Birkhauser, Basle, 1979, p. 60.
4. K. S. Squibb and R. J. Cousins, *Environ. Physiol. Biochem., 4*:24 (1974).
5. J. K. Piotrowski, B. Trojanowska, J. M. Wisniewsk-Knypl, and W. Bolanowska, *Toxicol. Appl. Pharmacol., 27*:11 (1974).
6. K. S. Squibb, R. J. Cousins, and S. L. Feldman, *Biochem. J., 164*:223 (1977).
7. I. Bremner and B. W. Young, *Biochem. J., 157*:517 (1976).
8. J. H. R. Kagi, S. R. Himoelhoch, P. D. Whanger, J. L. Bethune, and B. L. Vallee, *J. Biol. Chem., 249*:3537 (1974).
9. R. H. O. Bühler and J. H. R. Kagi, *FEBS Lett., 39*:229 (1974).
10. L. Rydén and H. F. Deutsch, *J. Biol. Chem., 253*:519 (1978).
11. B. L. Vallee in *Metallothionein* (J. H. R. Kagi and M. Nordberg, eds.), Birkhauser, Basle, 1979, p. 19.
12. J. D. Otvos and I. M. Armitage, *J. Amer. Chem. Soc., 101*:7734 (1979).
13. J. H. R. Kagi and B. L. Vallee, *J. Biol. Chem., 236*: 2435 (1961).
14. G. Sokolowski and U. Weser, *Hoppe-Seyler's Z. Physiol. Chem., 356*:1715 (1975).
15. Kojima, C. Berger, B. L. Vallee, and J. H. R. Kagi, *Proc. Natl. Acad. Sci. USA, 73*:3413 (1976).
16. H.-B. Bürgi, *Helv. Chim. Acta, 57*:513 (1974).
17. S. G. Shapiro, K. S. Squibb, L. A. Markowitz, and R. J. Cousins, *Biochem. J., 175*:833 (1978).
18. R. D. Andersen, W. P. Winter, J. J. Maher and I. A. Bernstein, *Biochem. J., 174*:327 (1978).
19. Y. Kojima, C. Berger, and J. H. R. Kagi in *Metallothionein* (J. H. R. Kagi and M. Nordberg, eds.) Birkhauser, Basle, 1979, p. 153.

20. I-Y. Huang, H. Tsunoo, M. Kimura, H. Nakashima, and A. Yoshida in *Metallothionein* (J. H. R. Kagi and M. Nordberg, eds.) Birkhauser, Basle, 1979, p. 169.

21. I. M. Armitage, R. T. Pajer, A. J. M. Schoot Uiterkamp, J. F. Chlebowski, and J. E. Coleman, *J. Amer. Chem. Soc., 98*:5710 (1976).

22. J. L. Sudmeier and S. J. Bell, *J. Amer. Chem. Soc., 99*:4499 (1977).

23. D. B. Bailey, P. D. Ellis, A. D. Cardin, and W. D. Behnke, *J. Amer. Chem. Soc., 100*:5236 (1978).

24. D. B. Bailey, P. D. Ellis, and J. A. Fee, *Biochemistry, 19*:591 (1980).

25. T. Drakenberg, B. Lindman, A. Cavé, and J. Parello, *FEBS Lett., 92*:346 (1978).

26. S. Forsén, E. Thulin, and H. Lilja, *FEBS Lett., 104*:123 (1979).

27. B. R. Bobsein and R. J. Myers, *J. Amer. Chem. Soc., 102*:2454 (1980).

28. J. D. Otvos and I. M. Armitage, *Biochemistry*, 19:4031 (1980).

29. I. M. Armitage, A. J. M. Schoot Uiterkamp, J. F. Chlebowski, and J. E. Coleman, *J. Magn. Reson., 29*:375 (1978).

30. R. A. Haberkorn, L. Que, Jr., W. O. Gillum, R. H. Holm, C. S. Liu, and R. C. Lord, *Inorg. Chem., 15*:2408 (1976).

31. J. D. Otvos and I. M. Armitage in *Metallothionein* (J. H. R. Kagi and M. Nordberg, eds.) Birkhauser, Basle, 1979, p. 249.

32. D. C. Jicha and D. H. Busch, *Inorg. Chem., 1*:872 (1962).

33. H. Shindo and T. L. Brown, *J. Amer. Chem. Soc., 87*:1904 (1965).

34. P. Strickler, *Chem. Commun.*:655 (1969).

35. J. D. Otvos and I. M. Armitage, unpublished results.

36. I. D. Campbell, C. M. Dobson, R. J. P. Williams, and P. E. Wright, *FEBS Lett., 57*:96 (1975).

37. R. Freeman and H. D. W. Hill in *Dynamic Nuclear Magnetic Resonance Spectroscopy* (L. Jackman and F.A. Cotton, eds.) Academic Press, 1975, p. 131.

38. R. Freeman and G. A. Morris, *Bull. Magn. Reson., 1*:5 (1979).

39. K. T. Suzuki, S. Takenaka, and K. Kubota, *Arch. Environm. Contam. Toxicol., 8*:85 (1979).

40. M. Vasak, *J. Amer. Chem. Soc., 102*:3953 (1980).

41. R. W. Olafson, R. G. Sim, and K. G. Boto, *Comp. Biochem. Physiol., 62*:407 (1979).

42. R. W. Olafson, A. Kearns, and R. G. Sim, *Comp. Biochem. Physiol., 62*:417 (1979).

43. K. Lerch and R. W. Olafson, *J. Biol. Chem.* (in press).

CHAPTER 5

LIGAND-DNA INTERACTIONS IN SOLUTION AROMATIC DICATION AND STEROID DIAMINE COMPLEXES

Dinshaw J. Patel
Department of Polymer Chemistry
Bell Laboratories
Murray Hill, New Jersey

The molecular basis of the pharmacological activity of drugs that interact with DNA is currently actively being pursued by structural studies in the crystalline state and conformational and dynamic investigations in solution [1-4]. This area of research has received considerable stimulus following the X-ray crystallographic solution at atomic resolution of several intercalation complexes involving planar ligands inserted into miniature dinucleoside duplexes [5-8]. These advances in the solid state are paralleled by high resolution Nuclear Magnetic Resonance (NMR) studies which have deduced structural and dynamic aspects of the complexes of intercalating, partial insertion and groove binding ligands with oligonucleotides and synthetic DNAs in solution [9-12].

Our laboratory has focussed its efforts on the application of NMR spectroscopy to investigate the structure and dynamics of nucleic acids at the oligomer [13] and synthetic DNA [11] level, as well as their complexes with antibiotics, mutagens and antitumor agents [11,13]. Two earlier reviews dealt with the duplex to strand transition of synthetic DNAs with an alternating inosine-cytidine [14], guanosine-cytidine [14] and adenosine-uridine [15] sequences and their complexes with the intercalating agents ethidium [14], terpyridine platinum [14], proflavine [15], and daunomycin [15] and the groove binding agent netropsin [15].

This review brings together the remainder of our recent research. It begins by describing the NMR parameters for poly(dI-⁵brdC) in low and high salt solution. This synthetic DNA is of considerable interest since it inverts its circular dichroism spectrum in high salt [16] and is a potential candidate for the salt dependent right-handed to left-handed helical conformational transition observed previously for $(dG-dC)_n$ in solution [17,16] and in the crystalline state [18].

We next evaluate in considerable detail the interaction of a nitrophenyl dication reporter molecule (custom synthesized by the late Professor E. Gabbay) and a steroid diamine with the synthetic DNA poly(dA-dT) in low salt. The aromatic ring of the reporter molecule is a potential intercalating agent while this mode is precluded to the nonplanar steroid diamine. An investigation of these complexes may help to establish the NMR parameters distinguishing full intercalation between stacked parallel base pairs and partial insertion between tilted base pairs at the binding site.

I. POLY(dI-5brdC) CONFORMATION IN LOW SALT

The NMR parameters of poly(dI-5brdC) have been monitored at the exchangeable protons in H_2O, the nonexchangeable base and sugar protons in ^2H_2O and the phosphate groups of the backbone. The results are compared with the NMR parameters for poly(dI-dC) published earlier [19] to determine the effect of the 5-bromo substituent on the cytidine ring.

1. Hydrogen Bonding

The integrity of the poly(dI-5brdC) duplex was probed by recording the exchangeable proton spectra in H_2O solution. The NMR resonances observed in the spectral region from 7 to 16 ppm are presented in Figure 1 with the exchangeable protons designated by asterisks.

Previous investigations have demonstrated that the imino exchangeable proton of nonterminal base pairs in nucleic acid duplexes are in slow exchange with solvent H_2O and resonate downfield from 11 ppm [20,21].

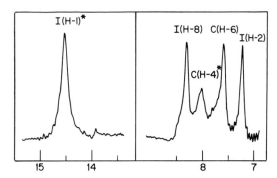

Figure 1. The 360 MHz proton NMR spectra of the exchangeable protons in poly(dI-^{5}brdC) in 0.1 M NaCl, 10 mM phosphate, 1 mM EDTA, 80% H_2O - 20% D_2O, pH 7.5 at 37°C. Spectrum A covers the spectral range 13.5 to 15.5 ppm with the inosine H-1 proton designated by an asterisk. Spectrum B covers the 7 to 9 ppm region with the cytidine 4 amino proton designated by an asterisk. No additional exchangeable resonances could be detected between 9 to 14 ppm and between 15 to 17 ppm.

The inosine H-1 imino proton is observed in poly(dI-^{5}brdC) at 14.53 ppm with a line width of 45 Hz at 37°C (Figure 1A) demonstrating formation of a base-paired duplex at this temperature.

An additional exchangeable resonance is observed amongst the nonexchangeable protons characteristic of the 7.0 and 8.5 ppm spectral region in the spectrum of poly(dI-^{5}brdC) in H_2O solution (Figure 1B). Previous studies on cytidine containing tetranucleotide duplexes have demonstrated that the hydrogen-bonded 4 amino proton resonates 1.0 to 1.5 ppm downfield from its exposed counterpart [22,23]. This permits the assignment of poly(dI-^{5}brdC) exchangeable resonance at 8.02 ppm (Figure 1B) to the bromocytidine 4-amino proton participating in a Watson-Crick hydrogen bond.

The chemical shifts of the Watson-Crick hydrogen-bonded imino and amino protons in poly(dI-dC) [19] and poly(dI-^{5}brdC) are compared in Table I. The 4-amino cytidine proton which is located adjacent to the 5-bromo substituent, shifts 0.65 ppm downfield on going from poly(dI-dC) to poly(dI-^{5}brdC). By contrast, the inosine H-1 proton shifts 0.55 ppm to higher field on 5-bromo substitution of the pyrimidine ring.

The temperature dependence of the chemical shifts of the exchangeable inosine H-1 and cytidine H-4 Watson-Crick base protons are compared with the corresponding parameters for the nonexchangeable inosine H-2, inosine H-8 and cytidine H-6 base protons of poly(dI-^{5}brdC) in the duplex

TABLE I

Chemical Shifts of the Hydrogen-Bonded Exchangeable Protons in Poly(dI-dC) and poly(dI-⁵brdC) in Solution

| | Watson-Crick proton shifts, ppm | |
	Inosine H-1	Cytidine H-4
Poly(dI-dC)[a](19)	15.15	7.40
Poly(dI-⁵brdC)[b]	14.61	8.05

[a] Buffer: 0.1 M phosphate, 1 mM EDTA, H_2O, 25°C
[b] Buffer: 0.1 M NaCl, 10 mM phosphate, 1mM EDTA, H_2O, 25°C

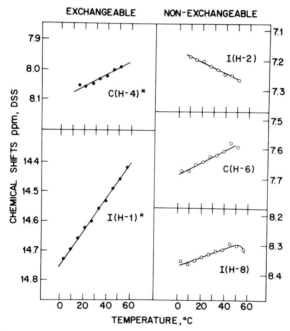

Figure 2. The temperature dependence of the chemical shifts of the exchangeable (inosine H-1 and cytidine H-4) protons and nonexchangeable (inosine H-8 and H-2 and cytidine H-6) protons of poly(dI-⁵brdC) in 0.1 M NaCl, 10 mM phosphate, 1 mM EDTA, H_2O, pH 7.5 in the premelting transition region (0° to 55°C).

state between 0 and 55°C (Figure 2). The exchangeable resonances of the synthetic DNA shift to high field with increasing temperature in the duplex state while shifts to both low and high field are observed at the nonexchangeable protons (Figure 2). The magnitude of the temperature dependent chemical shift change is similar for the exchangeable cytidine H-4 proton and the nonexchangeable protons but is significantly greater for the exchangeable imino H-1 proton (Figure 2).

The chemical shift of the inosine H-1 proton in the open state resonates several ppm upfield from its chemical shift in the duplex state [11]. The large upfield shift of this resonance with temperature (Figure 2) may reflect, in part, a weakening of the hydrogen bond in the duplex state with increasing temperature.

The line width of the exchangeable inosine H-1 proton is compared with the corresponding data for the nonexchangeable inosine H-8 proton for poly (dI-^{5}brdC) duplex state between 9 and 55°C (Figure 3). The inosine H-8 resonance in the synthetic DNA exhibits a line width of ~35 Hz between 55°C and 30°C and broadens to ~70 Hz on lowering the temperature to 0°C (Figure 3). The increase in line width reflects a shift in the equilibrium between branched and linear duplexes towards the latter with decreasing temperature [24-26].

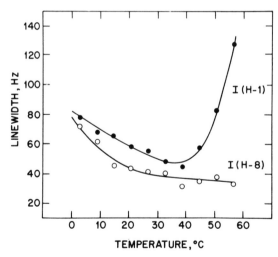

Figure 3. The temperature dependence of the line widths of the inosine H-1 exchangeable protons and the inosine H-8 nonexchangeable proton of poly(dI-^{5}brdC) in 0.1 M NaCl, 10 mM phosphate, 1 mM EDTA, H_2O, pH 7.5 in the premelting transition region (0° 55°C).

The exchangeable inosine H-1 resonance line width is broader by ~ 10 Hz compared with the inosine H-8 resonance line width between 0°C and 40°C (Figure 3). This reflects the contribution to the line width of the exchangeable resonance from the directly bonded ^{14}N quadrupolar nucleus. The inosine H-1 exchangeable resonance broadens dramatically between 45°C and 55°C (Figure 3). This observation requires a decrease in the lifetime of the hydrogen-bonded proton in the duplex state of the synthetic DNA at temperatures approaching the onset of the melting transition.

2. Duplex to Strand Transition

The nonexchangeable base and sugar protons of poly(dI-^{5}brdC) in 0.1 M NaCl have been recorded as a function of temperature in ^{2}H$_2$O solution and the temperature dependent chemical shifts are plotted in Figure 4. The base resonances can be readily assigned though it has not been possible to differentiate between the sugar protons linked to the inosine and bromocytidie rings. The base and sugar H-1' protons shift to high field on duplex formation, the sugar H-3' and H-5',5'' are less sensitive to the helix-coil transition while the H-2',2'' protons shift to both low and high field during the melting transition (Figure 4). The magnitudes of the upfield shifts on duplex formation are similar for poly(dI-^{5}brdC) (Figure 4) and those published previously for poly(dI-dC) [19]. The cytidine H-6 proton is most perturbed by the 5-bromo substitution at the adjacent position resulting in a 0.36 ppm downfield shift (Table II). Further, amongst the unassigned sugar H-1' protons, the resonance at lower field is perturbed to a greater extent on 5-bromo substitution of the cytidine ring of poly(dI-dC) (Table II).

The temperature dependent changes in the nonexchangeable proton shifts of poly(dA-^{5}brdU) in 0.1 M NaCl are plotted in Figure 5. These results provide a direct comparison between the synthetic DNAs, poly

TABLE II

Chemical Shifts of Poly(dI-dC) and Poly(dI-⁵brdC) in the Duplex State

| | Chemical shifts, δ d, ppm[a] | |
	Poly(dI-dC)[b]	Poly(dI-⁵brdC)[c]
I(H-8)	8.135	8.210
I(H-2)	7.315	7.230
C(H-6)	7.130	7.490
u(H-1')	5.540	5.510
d(H-1')	6.040	6.135

[a] The chemical shift in the duplex state, δ_d, is defined as the extrapolation of the temperature dependent premelting shift to its value at the transition midpoint.

[b] Buffer: 0.1 M phosphate, 1 mM EDTA, ^2H_2O, pH 7.0

[c] Buffer: 0.1 M NaCl, 10 mM phosphate, 1 mM EDTA, ^2H_2O, pH 7.3

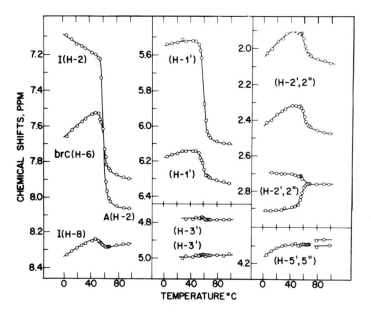

Figure 4. The temperature dependence (0° to 100°C) of the base and sugar proton chemical shifts of poly(dI-⁵brdC) in 0.1 M NaCl, 10 mM phosphate, 1 mM EDTA, ^2H_2O, pH 7.3.

(dI-⁵brdC) (Figure 4) and poly(dA-⁵brdU) (Figure 5) in aqueous solution.

3. Base Pair Overlaps

The upfield shifts at the base protons of poly(dI-⁵brdC) (Figure 4) and poly(dA-⁵brdU) (Figure 5) on duplex formation decrease in the order purine H-2 > bromopyrimidine H-6 > purine H-8 (Table III), similar to what has been previously reported for poly(dI-dC) (Table III) and poly (dA-dU) [14,15]. These upfield shifts on duplex formation reflect predominantly ring current contributions from nearest neighbor and next-nearest neighbor base pairs [27,28]. These results require that the synthetic DNAs poly(dA-dU), poly(dI-dC) and their 5-halogen substituted

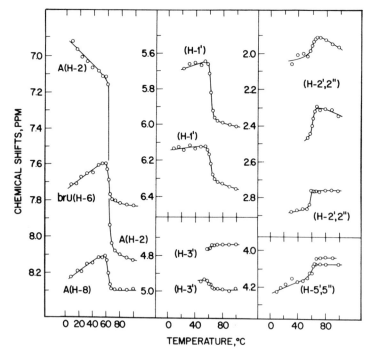

Figure 5. The temperature dependence (0° to 100°C) of the base and sugar proton chemical shifts of poly(dA-⁵brdU) in 0.1 M NaCl, 10 mM phosphate. 1 mM EDTA, ²H₂O.

TABLE III

Chemical Shift Change Associated with the Melting Transition of Poly(dI-dC) and Poly(dI-⁵brdC)

| | *Chemical shift change, $\Delta\delta$, ppm[a]* | |
	Poly(dI-dC)[b]	*Poly(dI-⁵brdC)[c]*
I(H-8)	0.107	0.082
I(H-2)	0.716	0.830
C(H-6)	0.402	0.383
u(H-1')	0.533	0.584
d(H-1')	0.208	0.176

[a] The duplex to strand transition chemical shift change, $\Delta\delta$, is defined as the chemical shift difference following extrapolation of the temperature dependent premelting and postmelting shifts to their values at the transition midpoints.

b Buffer: 0.1M phosphate, 1 mM EDTA, ^2H_2O, pH 7.0.

c Buffer: 0.1M NaCl, 10 mM phosphate, 1mM EDTA, ^2H_2O, pH 7.3.

pyrimidine analogs exhibit similar base pair overlap geometries in the duplex state.

4. Sugar Ring

We observe an interesting difference in the chemical shift changes at the upfield pair of sugar H-2',2" resonances associated with the melting transition of poly(dI-⁵brdC) and poly(dA-⁵brdU) in 0.1 M NaCl solution. These resonances shift to high field on poly(dI-⁵brdC) duplex formation (Figure 4) but to low field on poly(dA-⁵brdU) duplex formation (Figure 5). The origin of the structural basis for the sugar H-2',2" shift is not understood and so no clearcut explanation can be put forward for the observed differences between these two synthetic DNAs.

5. Duplex Dissociation Rates

Slow exchange between duplex and strand states of poly(dI-dC) resulted in doubling of the nonexchangeable proton spectra at temperatures corresponding to the melting transition [19]. By contrast, the exchange is intermediate on the NMR time scale for poly(dI-5brdC) since the extent of broadening is dependent on the chemical shift difference between duplex and strand states. Thus, the inosine H-8 proton, which exhibits a small melting transition chemical shift difference ($\Delta\delta = 0.08$ ppm), moves as an average resonance during the melting transition (Figure 4). The extent of broadening at the midpoint of the transition increases in the order: downfield H-1' < bromocytidine H-6, upfield H-1' < inosine H-2, which is exactly the order of increasing $\Delta\delta$ values. As an example, the limited data on the line width of the cytidine H-6 proton of poly(dI-5brdC) are plotted in Figure 6 and illustrate the large line width increase in the vicinity of the melting transition.

6.   Premelting Transition

A non-cooperative conformational change has been monitored by circular dichroism and polarographic techniques in natural and synthetic DNAs on lowering the temperature below the melting transition temperature region [29]. The transition has also been observed for poly(dA-dT) films by infrared dichroism and in solution by circular dichroism [30].

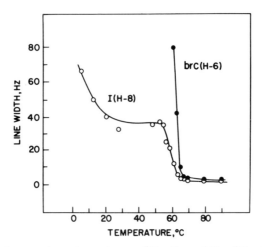

Figure 6. The temperature dependence of the line width of the inosine H-8 (o) and bromocytidine H-6 (o) protons of poly(dI-5brdC) in 0.1 M NaCl, 10 mM phosphate, 1 mM EDTA, ^2H_2O, pH 7.3.

The premelting transition is readily observed at the temperature dependent chemical shifts of the exchangeable and nonexchangeable base protons and the nonexchangeable sugar protons of poly(dI-^{5}brdC) in 0.1 M NaCl solution (Figures 2 and 4). The magnitude of the premelting change is most pronounced at the inosine H-1 proton, significant at the inosine H-8 and H-2, bromocytidine H-4 and H-6 protons and the upfield set of H-2′,2″ sugar protons, less pronounced at the H-1′ protons and not observed at the H-3′ protons and the downfield set of H-2′,2″ sugar protons (Figures 2 and 4). The inosine H-2 proton shifts to higher field on lowering the temperature in the premelting transition range while the remaining base and sugar resonances shift to lower field on decreasing the temperature.

These results suggest that the premelting conformational transition reflects (in part) changes in the base pair overlaps and the sugar phosphate backbone. We suggest that the structural basis of this transition may originate in the extent of propeller twisting of the base pairs [31-33] and/or unwinding of the double helix with temperature.

It is clear that the magnitude and direction of the premelting changes at the base positions (purine H-2, H-8 and pyrimidine H-6) are similar for poly(dI-^{5}brdC) Figure 4) and poly(dA-^{5}brdU) Figure 5), which indicates that this transition is independent of sequence in alternating purine (5-bromo) pyrimidine polynucleotide duplexes.

7. Phosphodiester Linkages

Previous ^{31}P NMR studies on poly(dA-dU), poly(dI-dC) [14] and poly(dG-dC) [34] in low salt demonstrated that the purine(3′-5′)pyrimidine and pyrimidine(3′-5′) purine phosphodiester linkages are unresolved at the synthetic DNA level. By contrast, resolved resonances separated by 0.25 ppm have been observed for 150 base pair (dA-dT)$_n$ [35] and resolved resonances separated by 0.2 to 0.5 ppm are observed for the synthetic RNAs poly(A-U), poly(I-C) [14] and poly(G-C) [34].

The proton noise decoupled ^{31}P spectrum of poly(dI-^{5}brdC) at 24°C and 45°C exhibits two partially resolvable resonances separated by ~0.23 ppm (Figure 7). The resonance to lower field exhibits the larger area and appears to be partially resolvable in the spectrum at 45°C (Figure 7). The observed chemical shift separation for the two ^{31}P resonances in poly(dI-^{5}brdC (Figure 7) is in contrast to the unresolved envelope observed for poly(dI-dC) under the same conditions [19].

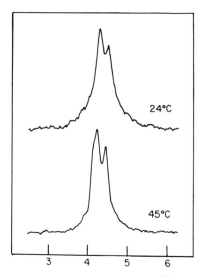

Figure 7. The proton noise decoupled 145.7 MHz ^{31}P NMR spectra of poly(dI-^{5}brdC) in 0.1 M NaCl, 10 mM cacodylate, 10 mM EDTA, ^{2}H$_2$O at 24°C and 45°C. The chemical shifts are upfield from the internal standard trimethylphosphate.

The observation of two ^{31}P resonances in the poly(dI-^{5}brdC) spectrum suggests that the brdCpdI and dIpbrdC phosphodiester linkages are distinct and probably reflect small variations in the O3'-P and P-O5' torsion angles about the gauche, gauche region. The origin of the unequal areas of the resolved ^{31}P resonances in the poly(dI-^{5}brdC) spectrum is not understood at this time.

8.   Summary

We have monitored the melting and premelting transitions of the synthetic DNA poly(dI-^{5}brdC) in low salt solution at the exchangeable hydrogen-bonded protons, the nonexchangeable base and sugar protons and the backbone phosphates as a function of temperature. The Watson-Crick inosine imino H-1 proton and the cytidine amino H-4 proton can be readily monitored in H$_2$O solution and provide markers for the integrity of the duplex state. The stacking of the base pairs in the double helix is reflected in the upfield shifts of the base protons on duplex formation. By contrast, the sugar H-1' chemical shifts predominantly monitor changes in the glycosidic torsion angles relating the base with the sugar ring. Two partially resolved resonances are observed in the proton noise decoupled ^{31}P spectrum of poly(dI-^{5}brdC) in low salt solution demonstrating small differences in the dIp^{5}brdC and ^{5}brdCpdI phosphodiester linkages in this halogen substituted synthetic DNA in aqueous solution. The premelting conformational transition is readily observable in poly(dI-^{5}brdC) and poly(dA-^{5}brdU) and is best monitored at the base protons and sugar H-2',2'' protons.

II. POLY(dI-^{5}brdC) CONFORMATION IN HIGH SALT

1. Salt Dependent Conformation

The seminal investigation of Pohl and Jovin demonstrated that (dG-dC)$_n$ oligomers and polymers underwent a cooperative and reversible structural transition in aqueous solution on addition of high salt [17] and high ethanol [36] concentrations. The characteristic inversion of the circular dichroism spectrum was also observed in mitomycin poly(dG-dC) complexes [37] while the antibiotic ethidium bromide cooperatively switched (dG-dC)$_n$ from the high salt to the low salt structure [38]. The transition was not detected in the ribo analog poly(G-C) or the corresponding synthetic DNAs poly(dA-dT), poly(dI-dC) and poly dG·poly dC on addition of high salt [17].

The high resolution ^1H and ^{31}P NMR studies of (dG-dC)$_n$ at the oligomer [16] and polymer [34] level demonstrated that every other glycosidic torsion angle, phosphodiester linkage and sugar pucker/orientation in high salt adopts a different conformation from that observed in B-DNA. These studies concluded that the symmetry unit repeats every base pair for (dG-dC)$_n$ in low salt but every two base pairs for (dG-dC)$_n$ in high salt solution [16].

These solution studies were complemented by the observation that crystals of the tetranucleotide (dC-dG)$_2$ underwent a structural transition with a change in the ionic strength of the medium [39]. Rich and coworkers have solved the structure of (dC-dG)$_3$ hexanucleotide duplex grown from a medium containing Na, Mg and polyamine cations [18]. They observed a left-handed double helical conformation with a zig-zag orientation of the deoxyribose-phosphate backbones. The symmetry repeat is every two base pairs with the guanosine residues adopting a *syn* glycosidic torsion angle and RNA type sugar pucker compared to an *anti* glycosidic torsion angle and DNA type sugar pucker at the cytidine residues [18]. The dGpdC and dCpdG phosphodiester linkages adopt different backbone O-P-O torsion angles in the crystalline state [18] and these results paralleled the observation of resolved ^{31}P resonances in the high salt spectra of (dG-dC)$_n$ in solution [16]. This left-handed conformation, designated Z-DNA, has also been observed in crystals of the (dC-dG)$_2$ tetranucleotide duplex [40,41].

It was of interest to determine whether the Z-DNA conformation could be adopted by alternating purine-pyrimidine sequences other than (dG-dC)$_n$ in aqueous solution. Thus, Arnott and coworkers have demonstrated that the characteristic fiber diffraction pattern for the Z-form of poly(dG-dC) was also observed for poly(dA-s^{4}dT) and poly(dA-dC)·poly(dG-dT) in the fiber state [42]. Klug and coworkers have proposed an alternating structure with a two base pair symmetry repeat for poly(dA-dT) [43] based on an X-ray analysis of pdA-dT-dA-dT in the crystalline state[44] and the observation that the nuclease DNAse I selectively cleaved alternating purine-pyrimidine synthetic DNAs at purine(3'-5')pyrimidine sites in contrast to cleavage at all sites in non-alternating natural DNA's in solution [45,46].

Klug and coworkers suggested that the generation of a DNA conformation with dinucleotide repeats for alternating purine-pyrimidine polynucleotides may be stabilized by introduction of halogen substituents at the pyrimidine 5 position [43]. We have therefore investigated the spectroscopic parameters for poly(dI-^{5}brdC) and poly(dA-^{5}brdU) as a function of salt in aqueous solution.

2. Circular Dichroism Studies

The circular dichroism spectra of poly(dI-^{5}brdC) in the presence of 0.1 M NaCl and 4.0 M NaCl between 220 nm and 340 nm are presented in Figure 8 [16]. We observed an inversion in the bands at $\sim$240 nm and $\sim$310 nm on addition of high salt with the transition exhibiting a midpoint at 3.3 M NaCl concentration [16]. By contrast, no such transition was observed in the C.D. spectrum of poly(dI-dC) on addition of high salt [17,47]. Thus, substitution of a polarizable substituent at the pyrimidine 5 position of poly(dI-dC) facilitates the formation of the alternating DNA conformation in high salt solution.

This observation cannot be extended to the related synthetic DNAs poly(dA-^{5}brdU) and poly(dA-^{5}idU) since their C.D. spectra did not invert as a function of salt.

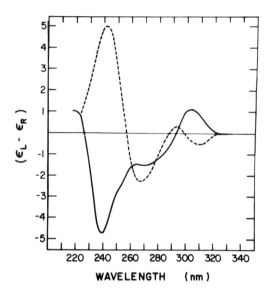

Figure 8. Circular dichroism spectra of poly(dI-⁵brdC) in 10 mM cacodylate, 1 mM EDTA, H_2O, pH 6.8 in the presence of 0.1 M NaCl (———) and 4.0 M (------).

3.   *31P NMR Studies*

Poly(dI-⁵brdC) and its sonicated fragments precipitate out of 4 M NaCl solution as a function of time at concentrations (mM) used in the NMR investigations. This prevented a systematic investigation of the NMR parameters for $(dI-^5brdC)_n$ duplex in high salt solution.

The synthetic DNAs poly(dG-dC) and poly(dI-⁵brdC) were sonicated to 150 ± 100 base pair fragments by Dr. Alfred Nordheim in Professor Alexander Rich's laboratory. Proton noise decoupled 145.7 MHz ³¹P NMR spectra were run on $(dG-dC)_n$ (Figures 9A, 9B) and $(dI-^5brdC)_n$ (Figures 9C, 9D) in the absence and presence of 4 M NaCl solution.

We observed resolved ³¹P resonances of roughly equal area separated by 1.5 ppm for $(dG-dC)_n$ in 4 M NaCl solution (Figure 9B). One set of peaks resonates between 4.0 and 4.3 ppm in the high salt spectrum (Figure 9B) similar to the chemical shift of $(dG-dC)_n$ in low salt (Figure 9A). The other resonance in high salt is a single peak shifted downfield to 2.8 ppm (Figure 9B) and corresponds to the altered phosphodiester grouping in the Z-DNA structure.

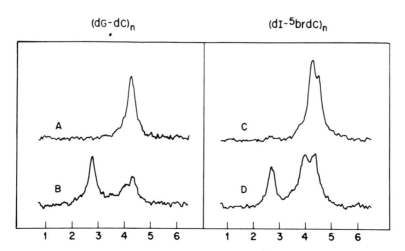

Figure 9. The proton noise decoupled 145.7 MHz ^{31}P NMR spectra of 150 base pair sonicated synthetic DNAs as a function of salt in 50 mM tris, 5 mM EDTA, ^2H_2O solution at 27°C. Spectra for (dG-dC)$_n$ in no added salt and 4 M NaCl are presented in (A) and (B), respectively. Spectra for (dI-^{5}brdC)$_n$ in no added salt and 4 M NaCl are presented in (C) and (D), respectively. The chemical shifts are upfield from internal standard trimethylphosphate.

We also observe resolved ^{31}P resonances separated by 1.5 ppm for (dI-^{5}brdC)$_n$ in 4 M NaCl solution (Figure 9D). However, the envelope of resonance centered about 4.2 ppm exhibits much greater intensity compared to the shifted resonance at 2.8 ppm (Figure 9D). The relative area of the shifted resonance decreases with increasing precipitation on standing of the (dI-^{5}brdC)$_n$ high salt solution.

The ^{31}P NMR results suggest that (dI-^{5}brdC)$_n$ can adopt (at least in part) the Z-DNA conformation where the symmetry unit repeats every two base pairs.

4. Summary

Previous NMR research from this laboratory demonstrated that (dG-dC)$_n$ adopts an alternating conformation in high salt solution for which the symmetry repeat is two base pairs [16]. This manifests itself in two ^{31}P resonances separated by 1.5 ppm with the downfield shifted resonance attributed to the altered phosphodiester linkage in the left-handed Z-DNA conformation observed in crystals of $(dC-dG)_3$ [18] and $(dC-dG)_2$ [40,41] and poly$(dG-dC)$ fibers [42]. The circular dichroism and ^{31}P NMR measurements presented above demonstrate that $(dI-^5brdC)_n$ but not $(dI-dC)_n$ can adopt the Z-DNA conformation in high salt solution. Thus, it appears that the left-handed zig-zag Z-DNA conformation is stabilized by polarizable substituents at the pyrimidine 5 position.

III. AROMATIC DIAMINE REPORTER MOLECULE · SYNTHETIC DNA COMPLEXES

The late Professor E. J. Gabbay synthesized a large series of reporter molecules to probe the interaction specificities of ligands with DNA [3]. These probes were utilized to investigate the criteria and steric requirements for full and partial intercalation complexes, the dissymmetric recognition of the helical sense of DNA and the sequence dependent dynamic structure of DNA in solution [3]. Various spectroscopic techniques including NMR spectroscopy were utilized to investigate these ligand-DNA complexes. The NMR spectral studies were of a preliminary nature since the investigators used natural DNA and did not observe the proton resonances of either the nucleic acid or the ligand in tightly bound complexes [3,48].

We report below on proton and phosphorus NMR studies of the interaction of nitroaniline labeled diammonium cations NP-I and NP-II [48] with poly$(dA-dT)$ in low salt buffer solution in an attempt to differentiate between partial and full intercalation of aromatic containing ligands into the synthetic DNA duplex.

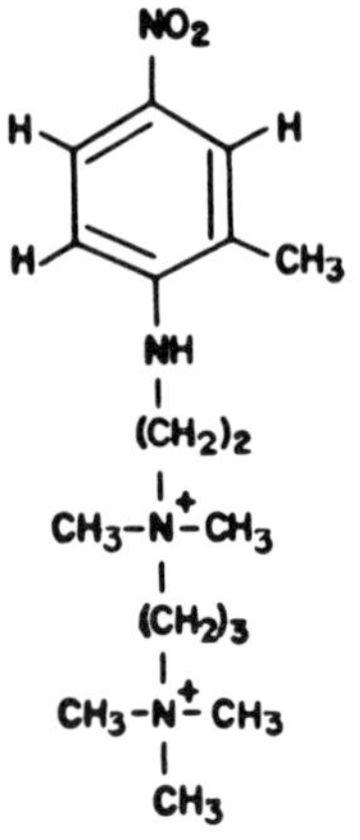

NP-I structure:

NO$_2$
H — ring — H
H — ring — CH$_3$
NH
(CH$_2$)$_2$
CH$_3$-N$^+$-CH$_3$
(CH$_2$)$_3$
CH$_3$-N$^+$-CH$_3$
CH$_3$

NP-II structure:

NO$_2$
H — ring — CH$_3$
H — ring — H
NH
(CH$_2$)$_2$
CH$_3$-N$^+$-CH$_3$
(CH$_2$)$_3$
CH$_3$-N$^+$-CH$_3$
CH$_3$

NP-I 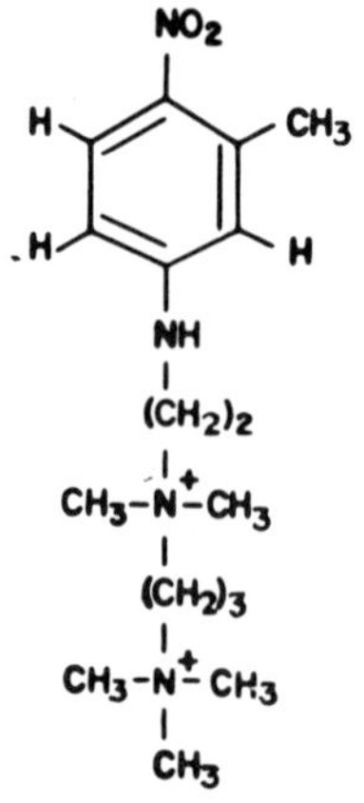   NP-II

We shall demonstrate that the resonances of the reporter molecule and the nucleic acid can be readily monitored in the complexes with the alternating purine-pyrimidine synthetic DNA poly(dA-dT) in contrast to the broadened out spectra observed with natural DNA. The studies were undertaken in 10 mM buffer solution in the absence of added salt in order to maximize the contributions of electrostatic interactions to the stability of the complex.

1. Hydrogen Bonding

The imino ring NH resonances in the Nuc/D=5 complexes of the reporter molecules NP-I and NP-II with poly(dA-dT) in 10 mM cacodylate buffer resonate at 12.93 ppm and 12.99 ppm, respectively, at 37°C (Figure 10). These results demonstrate that the base pairs are intact on complex formation and exhibit a chemical shift similar to what is observed in the synthetic DNA alone in solution.

We have followed the chemical shift and line width of this Watson-Crick hydrogen-bonded thymidine H-3 proton in the Nuc/D=5 NP-I·poly(dA-dT) complex as a function of pH at constant temperature and as a function of temperature at neutral pH. The exchangeable proton spectra for the complex between 11 and 14 ppm with increasing pH at 45°C are shown in Figure 11 and the chemical shifts and line widths summarized in Table IV. This imino proton can be detected between pH 6.5 and 9.0, exhibits a pH independent chemical shift of 12.93 ppm and broadens from ~130 Hz at pH 8.0 to ~230 Hz at pH 9.0 (Table IV). The pH dependence of the line width of the thymidine H-3 proton in the complex suggests that exchange

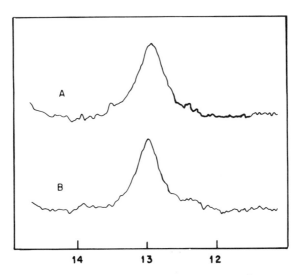

Figure 10.   The 360 MHz correlation proton NMR spectra (11 to 15 ppm) of (A) the NP-I·poly(dA-dT) complex, Nuc/D=5, and (B) the NP-II·poly(dA-dT) complex, Nuc/D=5 in 10 mM cacodylate, 1 mM EDTA, 80% H_2O - 20% ^2H_2O at 37°C. Spectra A and B were recorded at pH values of 7.05 and 6.75, respectively.

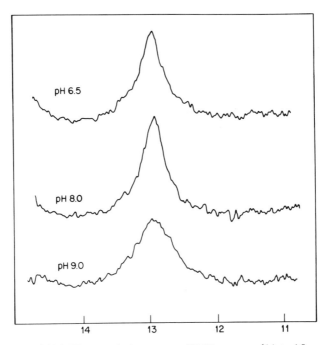

Figure 11.   The 360 MHz correlation proton NMR spectra (11 to 15 ppm) of the NP-I poly(dA-dT) complex, Nuc/D=5, in 10 mM cacodylate, 1 mM EDTA, 80% H_2O - 20% D_2O, 45°C, at pH 6.5, 8.0 and 9.0.

TABLE IV

Chemical Shifts and Line Widths of the Hydrogen-Bonded Exchangeable Protons in Nuc/D = 5 NP-I · Poly(dA-dT) Complex[a] as a Function of pH and Temperature

pH	Temperature (°C)	Chemical shift (ppm)	Line width (Hz)
6.5	45	12.93	140
8.0	45	12.92	133
9.0	45	12.93	233
6.5	45	12.93	140
6.5	55	12.865	121
6.5	65	12.80	190

[a] Buffer: 10 mM cacodylate, 1 mM EDTA, H_2O.

occurs by a pre-equilibrium pathway at 45°C by occasional leakage from the transiently open state with water [49-51,21].

The imino proton spectra of the complex at pH 6.5 between 45°C and 65°C are presented in Figure 12 and the spectral parameters summarized in Table IV. The thymidine H-3 Watson-Crick proton can be observed at 45°, 55° and 65°C (Table IV). The broadening of the resonance occurs with the onset of the melting transition (midpoint, $t_{1/2}$ = 71.5°C) as has been previously observed for poly(dA-dT) alone in solution [15].

The above results demonstrate the existence of a stable Watson-Crick imino hydrogen bond in the Nuc/D=5 NP-I·poly(dA-dT) complex in 10 mM buffer solution at temperatures corresponding to the premelting transition region.

2. Nonexchangeable Protons

The duplex to strand melting transition of the complexes of the reporter molecules NP-I and NP-II with poly(dA-dT) have been monitored at nonexchangeable base and sugar nucleic acid and reporter molecule protons as a function of temperature. Typical aromatic region spectra recorded in the vicinity of the melting temperature of these Nuc/D=5

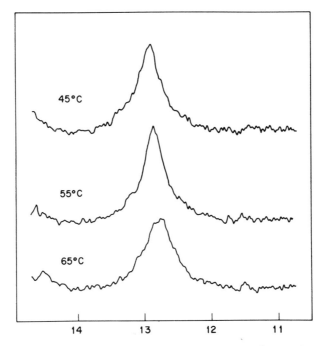

Figure 12. The 360 MHz correlation proton NMR spectra (11 to 15 ppm) of NP-
I·poly(dA-dT) complex, Nuc/D=5, in 10 mM cacodylate, 1 mM EDTA, 80%
H_2O - 20% D_2O, pH 6.5, at 45°, 55° and 65°C.

complexes are presented in Figure 13. The nitroaniline protons are designated by asterisks and are partially resolved from the nucleic acid resonances in the NP-I·poly(dA-dT) complex at 70.8°C (Figure 13A) and the
NP-II·poly(dA-dT) complex at 64.4°C (Figure 13B).

The 5 to 9 ppm nonexchangeable proton spectra of the NP-II·poly(dA-
dT), Nuc/D=5, in 10 mM buffer in the duplex state (59.9°C), during the
melting transition (65.4°C) and in the strand state (71.3°C) are presented
in Figure 14. The nucleic acid protons and the three aromatic protons on
the nitroaniline ring system (designated by asterisks) can be independently monitored as average resonances during the dissociation of the
complex with increasing temperature.

3. Reporter Molecule Resonances

We have monitored the nitroaniline ring protons and CH_3 groups in the
Nuc/D=5 complexes of the reporter molecules NP-I and NP-II with

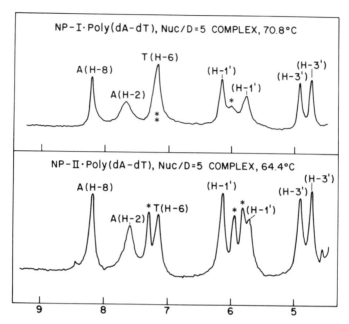

Figure 13. The 360 MHz proton NMR spectra (4.5 to 9 ppm) of (A) the Nuc/D=5 NP-I·poly(dA-dT) complex at 70.8°C and (B) the Nuc/D=5 NP-II·poly(dA-dT) complex at 64.4°C. The spectra were recorded in 10 mM cacodylate, 1 mM EDTA, ^{2}H$_2$O solution. These spectra were recorded at temperatures close to the transition midpoint for dissociation of the complex. The nitroaniline ring protons are designated by asterisks.

poly(dA-dT) in 10 mM cacodylate buffer as a function of temperature. The temperature dependent chemical shifts are plotted in Figure 15. The ring proton and CH$_3$ group resonances of NP-I and NP-II shift upfield on complex formation with the synthetic DNA. The upfield shifts are on the order of ~1.0 ppm at all four markers of the nitroaniline ring in the Nuc/D=5 NP-I·poly(dA-dT) complex and require that the reporter molecule intercalate between base pairs and the upfield shifts reflect ring current contributions from adjacent base pairs [27,28]. By contrast, the N-methyl resonances of the dication side chain are perturbed by ≤ 0.1 ppm and hence must lie in the groove of the DNA. The complex dissociates with a transition midpoint of 71.7± °C as monitored at the nitroaniline ring protons and represents stabilization of the poly(dA-dT) duplex by bound reporter molecule NP-I of 26.5°C.

The protons and CH$_3$ groups on the nitroaniline ring system of NP-II undergo somewhat smaller shifts of 0.7 to 0.9 ppm on formation of the

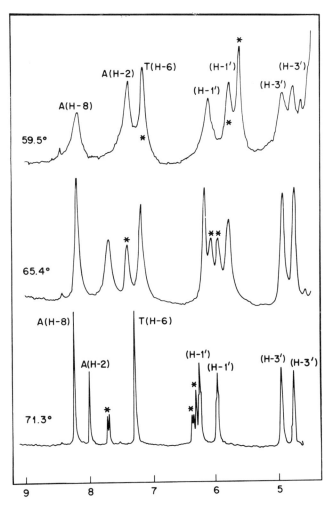

Figure 14. The 360 MHz proton NMR spectra (4.5 to 9 ppm) of the NP-II·poly(dA-dT) complex, Nuc/D=5, in 10 mM cacodylate, 1 mM EDTA, ^2H_2O at 59.5°, 65.4° and 71.3°C.

Nuc/D=5 poly(dA-dT) complex (Figure 15). The transition midpoint for complex dissociation is 66°C indicative of a 21°C stabilization by bound NP-II reporter molecule.

It should be noted that the nitroaniline protons of both reporter molecules shift as average peaks during the dissociation of the Nuc/D=5 poly(dA-dT) complexes indicative of fast exchange on the NMR time scale.

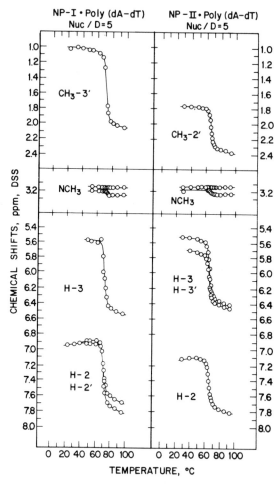

Figure 15. The temperature dependence of the nitrophenyl ring protons and methyl group and side chain N-methyl group chemical shifts in the NP-I·poly(dA-dT) complex, Nuc/D=5, and NP-II poly(dA-dT) complex, Nuc/D=5, in 10 mM cacodylate, 1 mM EDTA, ^2H_2O solution.

We have estimated the nitroaniline proton complexation shifts corresponding to the reporter molecule fully bound to the synthetic DNA by monitoring these chemical shifts as a function of the Nuc/D ratio at a fixed poly(dA-dT) concentration. The results for the nitroaniline CH_3 group in the NP-I·poly(dA-dT) complex as a function of the Nuc/D ratio are plotted in Figure 16. This CH_3 resonance exhibits a chemical shift of

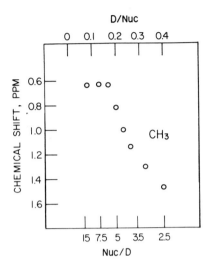

Figure 16. The chemical shift of the nitrophenyl ring CH_3 group in the NP-I·poly(dA-dT) complex in 10 mM cacodylate, 1 mM EDTA, ^2H_2O, 40°C as a function of the Nuc/D ratio at a fixed synthetic DNA concentration.

~0.63 ppm at Nuc/D ratios of $\geqslant 6$ in the NP-I·poly(dA-dT) complex. However, the CH_3 group shifts downfield towards its value in the free reporter molecule when the Nuc/D ratio decreases below 6, conditions under which the binding sites are saturated and the observed nitroaniline CH_3 chemical shift is an average of free and bound reporter molecules. These limiting chemical shifts corresponding to NP-I fully bound to poly(dA-dT) are summarized in Table V along with the complexation shifts measured relative to NP-I at high temperature. We observe upfield shifts of 1.4 to 1.7 ppm at all four positions of the nitroaniline ring system on formation of the poly(dA-dT) complex. The large magnitude of these upfield shifts at all four markers demonstrates full intercalation of the nitroaniline ring system between base pairs of the synthetic DNA. A partial insertion would have resulted in a different magnitude of the upfield shifts at positions 2,2' relative to the positions 3,3' which was not observed experimentally.

4.   Nucleic Acid Base Resonances

It is readily apparent from the spectra of the reporter molecule·poly(dA-dT) complexes in Figures 13 and 14 that the nucleic acid resonances are

TABLE V

Nitroaniline Ring Proton Complexation Shifts on Formation of the Nuc/D = 8 NP-I Poly(dA-dT) Complex[a]

	Free NP-I[b] (δ, ppm)	Nuc/D=8 Complex[c] (δ, ppm)	Upfield complexation shift[d] (Δδ, ppm)
H-2'	8.030	6.595	1.435
H-2	8.110	6.395	1.715
H-3	6.770	5.155	1.615
CH_3-3'	2.220	0.575	1.645

[a] Buffer: 10 mM cacodylate, 0.1 mM EDTA, ^2H_2O.

[b] 1 mM NP-I in 10 mM cacodylate, 0.1 mM EDTA, ^2H_2O at 82°C.

[c] NP-I Poly (dA-dT) complex, Nuc/D=8, in 10 mM cacodylate, 0.1 mM EDTA, ^2H_2O at 43.0°C.

[d] The upfield complexation shift is the difference between the chemical shift of the Nuc/D=8 complex at 43°C and free NP-I at 82°C.

not broadened beyond detection on complex formation. We have plotted the line width of the adenosine H-8 resonance in the Nuc/D=5 NP-I·poly(dA-dT) complex (Figure 17A) and the Nuc/D=5 NP-II·poly(dA-dT) complex (Figure 17B) in 10 mM cacodylate solution. We have therefore been able to monitor the nucleic acid resonances between 30° and 90°C through the dissociation of the nitroaniline reporter molecule ·poly(dA-dT) complexes (Figures 18 and 19).

The temperature dependent chemical shifts of the base protons of the Nuc/D=5 NP-I·poly(dA-dT) complex and the Nuc/D=5 NP-II·poly(dA-dT) complex are plotted in Figure 18 and are compared with the same parameters for poly(dA-dT) in 10 mM buffer solution. Formation of the reporter molecule synthetic DNA complexes results in downfield shifts of the adenosine H-2 and H-8 and the thymidine H-6 and CH_3-5 protons (Figure 18). The chemical shifts of the base protons in the Nuc/D=5 nitroaniline dication intercalation complexes reflect the net difference between the ring current contributions of the nitroaniline ring [52] and dA·dT base pair [27,28] it displaces as a result of intercalation. Since the ring current contributions are larger for the base pair, intercalation results in downfield shifts at the nucleic acid base resonances.

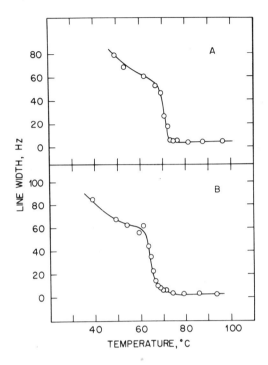

Figure 17. The temperature dependence of the line width of the adenosine H-8 resonance in (A) the Nuc/D=5 NP-I·poly(dA-dT) complex and (B) the Nuc/D=5 NP-II·poly(dA-dT) complex in 10 mM cacodylate, 1 mM EDTA, ^2H_2O solution.

5.   Nucleic Acid Sugar Resonances

The sugar H-1′ protons of poly(dA-dT) undergo small upfield shifts on formation of the nitroaniline dication reporter molecule complexes (Figure 19). Since the sugar H-1′ proton chemical shifts predominantly monitor variations in the glycosidic torsion angles [53], the results suggest small changes at these angles on formation of the intercalation site.

The nucleic acid base and sugar protons in the reporter molecule poly-(dA-dT) complex shift as average peaks during the melting transition (Figures 18 and 19) requiring that the dissociation kinetics be fast on the NMR time scale.

Poly(dA-dT)   NP-I·Poly(dA-dT) NP-II·Poly(dA-dT)

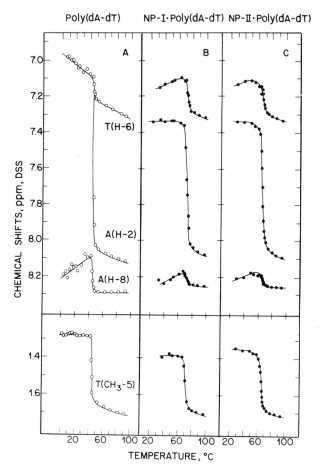

Figure 18. The temperature dependence of the base proton chemical shifts in (A) poly(dA-dT), (B) the Nuc/D=5 NP-I·poly(dA-dT) complex and (C) the Nuc/D=5 NP-II·poly(dA-dT) complex in 10 mM cacodylate, 1 mM EDTA, ^2H_2O solution.

6. *Phosphodiester Linkages*

The synthetic DNA poly(dA-dT) contains dApdT and dTpdA phosphodiester linkages which are not resolved at the polynucleotide level [11].

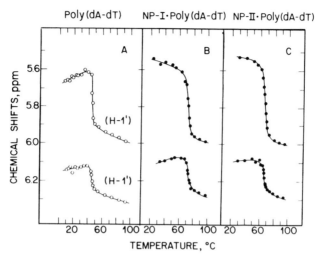

Figure 19. The temperature dependence of the sugar H-1' proton chemical shifts of (A) poly(dA-dT), (B) the Nuc/D=5 NP-I·poly(dA-dT) complex and (C) the Nuc/D=5 NP-II·poly(dA-dT) complex in 10 mM cacodylate, 1 mM EDTA, ^2H_2O solution.

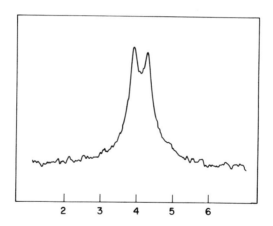

Figure 20. The proton noise decoupled 145.7 MHz ^{31}P NMR spectrum of the NP-I·poly(dA-dT) complex, Nuc/D=5, in 10 mM cacodylate, 10 mM EDTA, ^2H_2O solution at 52°C. The chemical shifts are upfield from internal standard trimethylphosphate.

However, recent studies on 150 base pair $(dA\text{-}dT)_n$ gave two resonances separated by 0.25 ppm in solution [35], and resolved peaks have also been observed for poly(dA-dT) fibers when the fiber axis is oriented parallel to the magnetic field [54].

The proton noise decoupled 145.7 MHz ^{31}P NMR spectrum of the Nuc/ D=5 NP-I·poly(dA-dT) complex in 10 mM cacodylate buffer at 52°C is shown in Figure 20. We observe two partially resolved resonances separated by 0.38 ppm and assign them to the dTpdA and dApdT phosphodiester groupings in the reporter molecule poly(dA-dT) complex. The observation of resolved resonances implies that the nitroaniline dication exhibits a sequence specificity in its complex with the alternating purine-pyrimidine synthetic DNA and shifts the phosphodiester linkage at the intercalation site to lower field. Since the two phosphate linkages cannot be assigned at this time we remain uncertain whether intercalation occurs at dTpdA or dApdT sites.

7. Summary

We have characterized the complexes of nitroaniline dication reporter molecules NP-I and NP-II with the synthetic DNA poly(dA-dT) by independently monitoring the ligand and nucleic acid resonances as average peaks during the temperature dependent dissociation of the complex. Base pairing is maintained on complex formation with the thymidine H-3 Watson-Crick proton readily observable up to pH 9 and at temperatures below ~65°C ($t_{1/2}$ of complex = 71.5°C).

The proton and methyl groups on the nitroaniline ring of NP-I shift upfield by 1.4 to 1.7 ppm on complex formation with poly(dA-dT), indicating full intercalation of the phenyl ring between base pairs. The nucleic acid base proton complexation shifts reflect the replacement of a base pair by the intercalating nitroaniline ligand while the sugar H-1' complexation shifts suggest small changes in the glycosidic torsion angles on generation of the intercalation site.

The observation of partially resolved dTpdA and dApdT ^{31}P resonances in the neighbor exclusion nitroaniline dication·poly(dA-dT) complex demonstrates that the phosphodiester O-P torsions are somewhat different at the intercalative and nonintercalative sites. These results also suggest that the nitroaniline reporter molecules intercalate either at pyrimidine (3'-5') purine or purine (3'-5') pyrimidine sites in the synthetic DNA with an alternating purine-pyrimidine sequence.

IV. STEROID DIAMINE · SYNTHETIC DNA COMPLEXES

Several lines of physicochemical, structural and theoretical evidence require considerable flexibility of the DNA double helix [55-62] as manifested in the folding of nucleic acids around histones in chromatin and the packaging of DNA in phage heads. Thus, it has been proposed that the DNA helix can fold by abrupt changes in the chain direction where the structural changes are localized at kink sites [63,64] or by smooth folding of the double helix where the structural changes are distributed along the chain [65,66,59]. These concepts have been extended by Sobell who suggests that the kink is a key intermediate in the process of drug intercalation into DNA and that the base pairs are kinked at the ligand binding site in steroid diamine-nucleic acid complexes [67].

Steroid diamines bind to DNA in low salt solution with saturation occurring at one molecule bound per five nucleotides, corresponding to the neighbor exclusion model for complex formation [68-70]. Sedimentation studies demonstrate that the steroid diamine unwinds covalently circular superhelical DNA to half the extent on a molar basis as the ethidium bromide intercalative complex [71-73].

The importance of electrostatic interactions to the stability of the complex is demonstrated by the dependence of the binding free energy on salt concentration [74,75]. The DNA double helix undergoes a conformational change on complex formation in solution as demonstrated by changes in the hydrodynamic, circular dichroism, transient electric field dichroism and nuclear magnetic resonance parameters [76,77,34].

Since the steroid diamine is non-planar it cannot intercalate between the base pairs of the duplex. Waring and Henley have investigated the binding of a series of stereoisomeric quarternary diaminoandrostanes by monitoring the viscosity and sedimentation properties of their DNA complexes [73]. They observe strong binding of the 3β, 5α, 17β stereoisomer (dipyrandium) with the preferred α stereochemistry at position 5 of the A/B ring juncture and β stereochemistry at the quaternary substitutions at positions 3 and 17 [73].

High resolution NMR spectroscopy can be used to probe the structural and dynamic aspects of nonintercalative drug-nucleic acid complexes, and hence studies were undertaken on the interaction of the steroid diamine dipyrandium and the synthetic DNA poly(dA-dT) as a function of Nuc/D ratio in aqueous solution [77]. The NMR parameters of the proton markers on the base and sugar rings of the polynucleotide, as well as the steroid diamine, can be independently monitored through the temperature dependent melting transition. The NMR studies were undertaken in the absence of added salt to maximize the electrostatic contributions to the stability of the complex.

1. Steroid Diamine Stabilization of the Duplex

The effect of the dipyrandium on the thermal melting transition of poly(dA-dT) can be readily monitored at the nucleic acid 260 nm absorption band in the complex. Typical differential melting curves for the dipyrandium·poly(dA-dT) complex in 10 mM buffer at Nuc/D ratios ranging from 50:1 to 1:1 are plotted in Figure 21. The steroid diamine stabilizes the thermal transition of the synthetic DNA (0.15 mM in nucleotides) with the transition midpoint increasing from 42.5°C in poly(dA-dT) to 59.0°C in the Nuc/D=5 complex in 10 mM buffer solution (Figure 21).

2. Steroid Diamine Binds in the Minor Groove

It should be possible to differentiate between ligand binding to the minor and major grooves of DNA by introduction of bulky substituents on the base pair edges. This can be readily undertaken by studying 5-halopyrimidine substituted synthetic DNAs in which the bulky substituent is located in the major groove.

The stabilization of the synthetic DNAs poly(dA-dU), poly(dA-^{5}brdU) and poly(dA-^{5}idU), as well as poly(dI-dC) and poly(dI-^{5}brdC) by bound dipyrandium at a Nuc/D=5 ratio in 10 mM buffer are summarized in Table VI. There is somewhat greater stabilization by bound dipyrandium of the 5-halogen substituted synthetic DNAs compared with their unsubstituted analogs (Table VI). These results which suggest that the steroid diamine binds to the minor groove are supported by a previous observation by Saucier that spermine (which binds in the minor groove) and steroid diamines bind competitively to DNA [74].

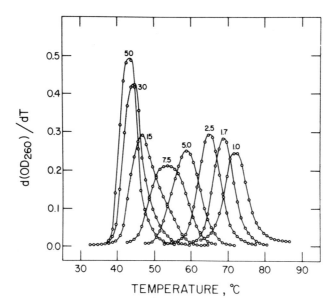

Figure 21.   The 260 nm ultraviolet-visible absorbance melting curves (first heating cycle) in differentiated form of poly(dA-dT) and the dipyrandium·poly(dA-dT) complexes, Nuc/drug = 50 to 1, in 10 mM cacodylate buffer, 1 mM EDTA, H_2O, pH 5.3. The poly(dA-dT) concentration was fixed at 0.15 mM. The melting curves were run on a Gilford 2400-2 spectrophotometer equipped with a thermoelectric device, a thermoprogrammer and a reference compensator. The samples (0.25 cc) were heated at a constant rate of 1°C/min from 25° to 98°C. At the end of the run, the samples were cooled down to 25°C and subjected to a second heating cycle. No differences were observed between heating cycles.

TABLE VI

Stabilization[a] of Synthetic DNA Duplexes on Formation of Nuc/D = 5 Dipyrandium Complexes in 10 mM Buffer Solution

Synthetic DNA[b,c]	Δt_m °C[d]
Poly(dA-dU)	21.5°
Poly(dA-^{5}brdU)	26°
Poly(dA-^{5}idU)	30°
Poly(dI-dC)	15°
Poly(dI-^{5}brdC)	20.5°

[a] 260 nm absorbance melting curves (first heating cycle).

[b] Synthetic DNA concentration was fixed at 0.15 mM.

[c] 10 mM cacodylate buffer, 1 mM EDTA, H_2O, pH 5.3.

[d] Δt_m represents the stabilization of the transition midpoint of the synthetic DNA on formation of the Nuc/D=5 complex in 10 mM buffer solution.

3. Hydrogen Bonding

The stability of the Watson-Crick hydrogen bonds and their accessibility to solvent in poly(dA-dT) and the Nuc/D=5 dipyrandium·poly(dA-dT) complex in 25 mM buffer have been probed by monitoring the thymidine H-3 proton as a function of pH and temperature.

The imino proton spectra (11.5 to 14.5 ppm) of the Nuc/D=5 dipyrandium·poly(dA-dT) complex in 25 mM buffer have been recorded as a function of pH at 20.3°C (Figure 22). The Watson-Crick thymidine H-3 proton can be observed at 13.08 ppm in the complex at neutral pH with a line width of 170 Hz (Table VII) in contrast to a much narrower resonance with a line width of 80 Hz in the synthetic DNA in the absence of steroid diamine (Table VIII). This imino proton is also observed in the pH 8.0 spectrum of the dipyrandium complex but broadens out in the pH 8.8 spectrum at 20.3°C (Figure 22 and Table VII). By contrast, the imino proton can be readily observed for poly(dA-dT) between pH 7 and 8.75 under the same conditions (Table VIII).

These results demonstrate that the base pairs are intact at the steroid diamine binding site on the synthetic DNA. However, the larger line width of the thymidine H-3 proton and its susceptibility to base catalysis in the complex suggest that the base pairs are partially exposed to solvent at the steroid diamine binding site.

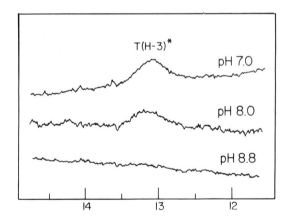

Figure 22. The 360 MHz continuous wave proton NMR spectra (11.5 to 14.5 ppm) of the dipyrandium·poly(dA-dT) complex, Nuc/D=5, in 25 mM cacodylate, 0.25 mM EDTA, H_2O 20.3°C, at pH 7.0, 8.0 and 8.8. The chemical shifts are referenced relative to internal standard TSP.

TABLE VII

Chemical Shifts and Line Widths of the Hydrogen-Bonded Exchangeable Protons in the Nuc/D = 5 Dipyrandium · Poly(dA-dT) Complex[a] as A Function of pH and Temperature

pH	Temperature (°C)	Chemical shift (ppm)	Line width (Hz)
7.0	20.3	13.08	170
8.0	20.3	13.16	195
8.8	20.3	too broad	
7.0	31.6	12.97	156
7.0	43.0	12.85	224
7.0	54.4	too broad	

[a] 25 mM cacodylate, 0.25 mM EDTA, H_2O. Transition midpoint, t_m = 77°C.

TABLE VIII

Chemical Shifts and Line Widths of the Hydrogen-Bonded Exchangeable Protons in Poly(dA-dT)[a] as a Function of pH and Temperature

pH	Temperature (°C)	Chemical shift (ppm)	Line width (Hz)
7.15	31.6	13.03	82
8.15	31.6	13.05	93
8.75	31.6	13.02	100
7.15	20.3	13.09	140
7.15	31.6	13.03	82
7.15	43.0	12.95	138

[a] Buffer: 25 mM cacodylate, 2.5 mM EDTA, H_2O. Transition midpoint, t_m = 45°C.

The imino proton spectral region in the Nuc/D=5 dipyrandium complex in 25 mM buffer has also been recorded at neutral pH as a function of temperature. The thymidine H-3 proton can be readily observed at 31.6°C and 43.0°C but this exchangeable resonance broadens out at 54.4°C (Figure 23) even though the transition midpoint as monitored by the nonexchangeable resonances is 77°C. Thus, the imino proton in the steroid diamine complex broadens out much below the onset of the thermal melting transition (t_m = 77°C) (Table VII) in contrast to the corresponding data for poly(dA-dT) in 25 mM buffer where the imino resonance broadens within a few degrees of the melting transition (t_m = 45°C (Table VIII).

The pH and temperature dependence of the thymidine H-3 proton in the neighbor exclusion steroid diamine·poly(dA-dT) complex is more characteristic of base pairs at the end (rather than the interior) of short DNA duplexes. We have previously demonstrated that fraying from the ends of DNA oligomer duplexes accounts for the sequential pH and temperature dependent line broadening of the imino protons of terminal base pairs [13].

4.   Thermal Dissociation of Complex

The exchangeable 6-amino adenosine and nonexchangeable base protons are readily observable in the aromatic spectral region (6 to 9 ppm) of the

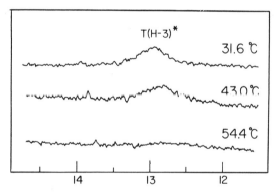

Figure 23. The 360 MHz continuous wave proton NMR spectra (11.5 to 14.5 ppm) of the dipyrandium·poly(dA-dT) complex, Nuc/D=5, in 25 mM cacodylate, 0.25 mM EDTA, H_2O, pH 7.0, at 31.6°C, 43.0°C and 54.4°C. The chemical shifts are referenced relative to internal standard TSP.

Nuc/D = 5 dipyrandium·poly(dA-dT) complex at neutral pH and 31.6°C (Figure 24). The nonexchangeable base resonances are well resolved in the neighbor exclusion complex, and hence it should be feasible to monitor the dissociation of the complex as a function of temperature in ^2H_2O solution.

The thermal transition of the complex can be monitored at the line widths or chemical shifts of individual resonances in the synthetic DNA and the steroid diamine. Typical line width data for the adenosine H-8 resonance during the thermal dissociation of the Nuc/D = 11.5 and Nuc/D = 5 complexes in 10 mM buffer are plotted in Figures 25A and 25B, respectively. The line widths narrow to ~75 Hz (55°C) with the onset of the thermal dissociation of the Nuc/D = 11.5 complex (Figure 25A) and to 35 Hz (65°C) for the Nuc/D = 5 complex (Figure 25B). These widths in the duplex state are much too broad to observe coupling constants of ≤10 Hz and hence the analysis has focussed on the chemical shift parameters.

The temperature dependent chemical shift of the adenosine H-2 resonance of poly(dA-dT) and its Nuc/D = 11.5, 5 and 3.5 dipyrandium complexes in 10 mM buffer are plotted in Figure 26. The adenosine H-2 resonance shifts as an average peak during the premelting and melting transition of the complexes. The bound dipyrandium stabilizes the poly(dA-dT) (17 mM in nucleotides) as reflected in the transition midpoint which increases from 45.0°C in the synthetic DNA to 74.5°C and 79.5°C for the Nuc/D = 5 and 3.5 complexes in 10 mM buffer solution (Figure 26). A biphasic melting transition is observed at a Nuc/D = 11.5 ratio with the lower and higher temperature transitions monitoring the opening of steroid-free base pair regions and those centered about bound dipyrandium, respectively (Figure 26).

5. Base Pair Overlap Geometries

The adenosine H-2 chemical shift in the duplex state of the synthetic DNA undergoes a dramatic downfield shift with increasing dipyrandium concentration (Figure 26). Further, downfield complexation shifts are also observed at the adenosine H-8, thymidine H-6 and CH_3-5 resonances in the Nuc/D = 11.5 and 5 steroid diamine complexes (Figure 27). Since the base proton chemical shifts are associated with the distance dependent ring current contributions [27,28], the downfield complexation shifts require a reduction of the stacking interactions between adjacent base pairs at the steroid diamine binding site.

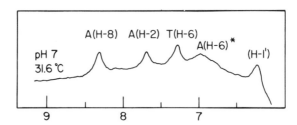

Figure 24. The 360 MHz continuous wave proton NMR spectrum (6.0 to 9.0 ppm) of the dipyrandium·poly(dA-dT) complex, Nuc/D=5, in 25 mM cacodylate, 0.25 mM EDTA, H_2O, pH 7 at 31.6°C. The exchangeable adenosine H-6 resonance is designated by an asterisk. The chemical shifts are referenced relative to internal standard TSP.

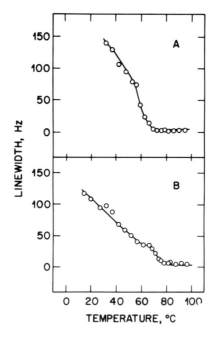

Figure 25. The temperature dependence of the line width of the adenosine H-8 resonance in the dipyrandium·poly(dA-dT) complex in 10 mM cacodylate, 0.1 mM EDTA, ^2H_2O solution. Plot A corresponds to the Nuc/D=11.5 complex, while plot B corresponds to the Nuc/D=5 complex.

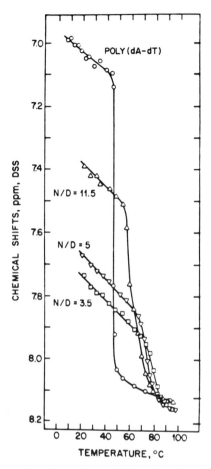

Figure 26. The temperature dependence of the adenosine H-2 resonance (7.0 to 8.2 ppm) for poly(dA-dT) and the dipyrandium·poly(dA-dT) complexes, Nuc/ D=11.5 , 5 and 3.5 in 10 mM cacodylate, 0.1 mM EDTA, ^2H_2O solution. The chemical shifts are relative to internal standard DSS.

6. *Premelting Transition*

The magnitude and direction of the temperature dependent premelting transition change at the adenosine H-2 resonance remains unchanged on addition of the steroid diamine to the synthetic DNA (Figure 26). The premelting change may reflect unwinding of the base pairs, a change in the

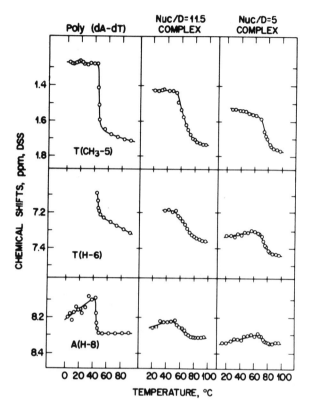

Figure 27. The temperature dependence of the nucleic acid base proton chemical shifts in poly(dA-dT) and the Nuc/D=11.5 and Nuc/D=5 dipyrandium poly (dA-dT) complexes in 10 mM cacodylate, 0.1 mM EDTA, ^2H_2O solution.

base pair twist and/or degree of branching with temperature. It is noteworthy that the steroid diamine does not perturb this conformational change.

7. Glycosidic Torsion Angle Change

The sugar H-1' chemical shifts are sensitive to changes in the glycosidic torsion angle linking the base and sugar rings [53]. The two sugar H-1' resonances of the synthetic DNA are perturbed on steroid diamine complex formation (Figure 28), which suggests a conformational change at both glycosidic torsion angles on formation of the dipyrandium·poly(dA-dT) complex. Indeed, the premelting conformational change monitored by the upfield H-1' resonance reverses direction in the steroid diamine complex (Figure 28).

8. Steroid Diamine Complexation Shifts

The temperature dependent chemical shifts of the steroid diamine protons and CH_3 groups in the Nuc/D = 11.5 and 5 dipyrandium·poly(dA-dT) complexes in 10 mM buffer are plotted in Figures 29 and 30, respectively. The steroid diamine resonances shift to high field as average peaks on complex formation (Figures 29 and 30) indictive of rapid exchange of the steroid diamine amongst potential nucleic acid binding sites on the NMR time scale at 10 mM ionic strength.

The magnitude of the upfield shifts are larger at the steroid diamine ring CH_3 groups compared to the side chain NCH_3 groups (Table IX, Figure 30). Several unassigned ring protons (Figure 29) exhibit upfield shifts which are larger than those observed for the CH_3 resonances (Figure 30).

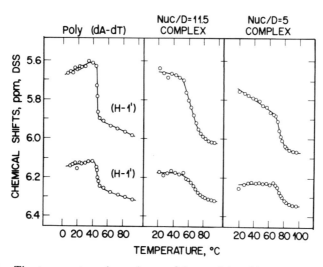

Figure 28. The temperature dependence of the nucleic acid sugar proton chemical shifts in poly(dA-dT) and the Nuc/D = 11.5 and Nuc/D = 5 dipyrandium·poly(dA-dT) complexes in 10 mM cacodylate, 0.1 mM EDTA, ^2H_2O solution.

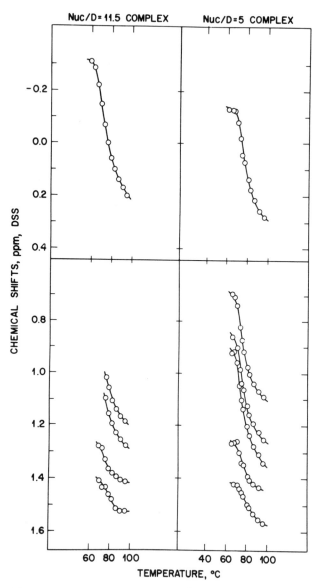

Figure 29. The temperature dependence of the resolvable steroid diamine proton chemical shifts in the Nuc/D=11.5 and Nuc/D=5 dipyrandium·poly(dA-dT) complexes in 10 mM cacodylate, 0.1 mM EDTA, ^2H_2O solution. Shifts are upfield from internal standard trimethylphosphate.

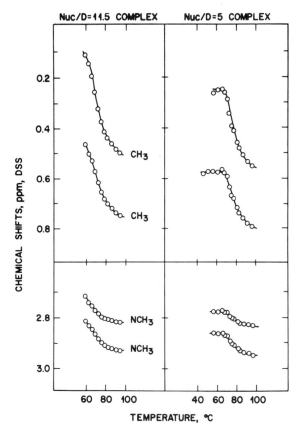

Figure 30. The temperature dependence of the steroid diamine CH_3 chemical shifts in the Nuc/D=11.5 and Nuc/D=5 dipyrandium·poly(dA-dT) complexes in 10 mM cacodylate, 0.1 mM EDTA, ^2H_2O solution.

9. *Steroid Diamine Insertion Between Tilted Base Pairs*

We demonstrated above that the nucleic acid nonexchangeable base protons of poly(dA-dT) shift to low field on complex formation with the steroid diamine (Figures 26 and 27) indicative of destacking of the base pairs at the binding site. By contrast, several proton and both CH_3 groups of the steroid diamine shift upfield on complex formation with poly(dA-

TABLE IX

Steroid Diamine CH₃ and NCH₃ Complexation Shifts on Formation of the Nuc/D = 11.5 Dipyrandium Poly(dA-dT) Complex[a]

	Free dipyrandium[b] (δ, ppm)	Nuc/D = 11.5 complex[c] (δ, ppm)	Upfield complexation shift[d] $(\delta \triangle, ppm)$
CH_3	0.82	~0.10	~0.72
CH_3	1.01	~0.46	~0.55
NCH_3	2.865	~2.71	~0.155
NCH_3	3.005	~2.81	~0.195

[a] Buffer: 10 mM cacodylate, 0.1 mM EDTA, ^2H_2O.

[b] 4.5 mg/ml dipyrandium in 10 mM phosphate, $2H_2O$ solution.

[c] Dipyrandium·Poly(dA-dT) complex, Nuc/D = 11.5, in 10 mM cacodylate, 0.1 mM EDTA, ^2H_2O at 60°C.

[d] The upfield complexation shift is the difference between the chemical shift of the Nuc/D = 11.5 complex at 60°C and free dipyrandium.

dT) (Figures 29 and 30) indicative of their location above the nucleic acid base pair planes.

The steroid diamine is nonplanar and hence it cannot fully insert between extended base pairs while spanning the backbone phosphates through its charged ends. Our NMR data are consistent with partial insertion of the steroid diamine between tilted base pairs at the complexation site. The ambiguities in the spectral assignments of the resolved steroid diamine protons and our inability to estimate the location (dT-dA or dA-dT) and magnitude of the tilt at the binding site from the NMR parameters make it premature to propose detailed models of the structure of the complex.

10. Steroid Diamine Binding to Strand State

We have observed that the chemical shifts of the proton and methyl groups of the steroid diamine in the dipyrandium poly(dA-dT)·complex at high temperature following completion of the duplex to strand transition are upfield from the corresponding values for dipyrandium alone in solution (Figure 31). This demonstrates that the steroid diamine also binds to and stacks over bases in the strand state in the post melting transition region. This conclusion also follows from the observed differences of the nucleic acid base proton chemical shifts of the synthetic DNA and its Nuc/D=5 complex at 95°C (Figure 27).

11. Sugar-Phosphate Backbone

The proton noise decoupled ^{31}P NMR spectra of poly(dA-dT) and the Nuc/D=5 dipyrandium·poly(dA-dT) complex in 10 mM cacodylate buffer at 30°C are presented in Figures 32A and 32B, respectively. The ^{31}P

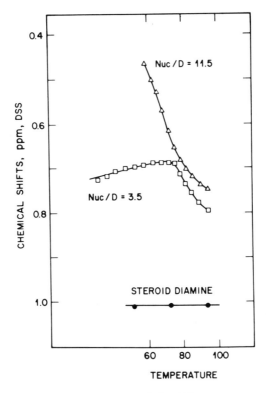

Figure 31. The temperature dependence of the CH_3 resonance in dipyrandium, the Nuc/D=11.5 and the Nuc/D=3.5 dipyrandium·poly(dA-dT) complex in 10 mM cacodylate, 0.1 mM EDTA, ^2H_2O solution.

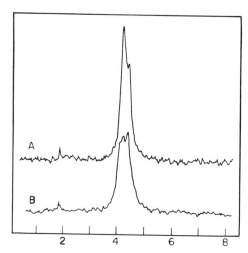

Figure 32. The proton noise decoupled 145.7 MHz ^{31}P NMR spectrum of (A) poly(dA-dT) in 10 mM cacodylate, 0.1 mM EDTA, ^{2}H$_2$O, pH 6.85, 29.5°C. (B) the Nuc/D=5 dipyrandium·poly(dA-dT) complex in 10 mM cacodylate, 0.1 mM EDTA, ^{2}H$_2$O, pH 6.85, 31°C. The chemical shifts are upfield from standard trimethylphosphate.

chemical shifts of the unresolved envelope in the synthetic DNA and its steroid diamine complex differ by < 0.1 ppm in the duplex state between 20°C and 40°C (Figure 32), and this suggests that the phosphodiester O-P torsion angles ω,ω' do not change significantly on generation of the steroid diamine binding site.

The ^{31}P NMR spectra of nucleosome core particles do not exhibit resolved ^{31}P resonances in either direction of the main phosphodiester peak at ~4.2 ppm upfield from standard trimethylphosphate [78-82]. These results do not rule out kinks in the DNA of the chromatin core particles as suggested by several authors [78-81] since we observe no shifts in the ^{31}P spectra of the kinked steroid diamine·synthetic DNA complex (Figure 32).

12. Summary

We have used NMR to probe structural and kinetic aspects of the binding of a nonintercalative steroid diamine to a synthetic DNA in solution. The exchangeable thymidine imino proton chemical shifts and line widths in the neighbor exclusion dipyrandium·poly(dA-dT) complex demonstrate that the base pairs are intact at the steroid diamine binding site. The observed downfield shifts of the base protons on complex formation are indicative of unstacking of base pairs with the steroid diamine partially inserting between tilted base pairs as reflected in the upfield complexation shifts of proton and methyl groups of the ligand. The NMR line shape parameters are consistent with fast exchange of the steroid diamine amongst potential binding sites. The similarity in the ^{31}P chemical shifts in the duplex state of poly(dA-dT) and its neighbor exclusion dipyrandium complex suggests that changes in the phosphodiester torsion angles do not occur on generation of the steroid diamine binding site.

V. CONCLUSION

We have demonstrated that synthetic DNA's with an alternating purine-pyrimidine sequence exhibit well resolved proton spectra in the duplex state and can be monitored as average peaks during the non-cooperative premelting and cooperative melting transitions. This review has focussed on poly(dI-^{5}brdC), and our research has demonstrated that this synthetic DNA changes its conformation from a helix with a symmetry repeat every base pair in low salt to a helix with a two base pair repeat in high salt solution.

We have compared the NMR parameters of the poly(dA-dT) complexes with a planar aromatic diamine and a non-planar steroid diamine in low salt solution. The nonexchangeable proton resonances of the ligand and the DNA can be monitored at various positions on each component and can be independently followed during the thermal dissociation of the complex.

The pH and temperature dependence of the line width of the Watson-Crick thymidine imino proton in these dication ligand-synthetic DNA complexes permits differentiation between full intercalation of the nitroaniline ring between parallel base pairs and partial insertion of the steroid ring between tilted base pairs at the binding site. The NMR parameters for the thymidine H-3 exchangeable resonances at the binding site in an intercalative complex are characteristic of a base pair in the interior of a duplex while this imino proton at the complexation site involving tilted base pairs exhibits the characteristics observed for terminal base pairs in oligonucleotide duplexes.

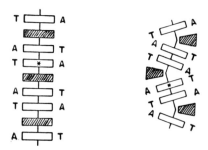

The nucleic acid proton complexation shifts are sensitive indicators of base pair unstacking on complex formation while the ligand resonances provide structural information on overlap geometries between ligand and base pairs at the binding site. The large (1.5 to 1.7 ppm) upfield shifts of the aromatic proton and methyl resonances on full intercalation of the nitroaniline ring between base pairs are to be compared with the smaller upfield shifts associated with partial insertion of the steroid diamine between base pairs.

These results demonstrate that proton NMR should be extremely useful in differentiating between full intercalation and partial insertion of aromatic amino acid side chains between base pairs in protein-DNA complexes.

We have demonstrated that ^{31}P NMR spectroscopy is a powerful probe for monitoring the sugar-phosphate backbone in DNA and ligand·DNA complexes in solution. Specifically, resolved ^{31}P resonances separated by 1.5 ppm are observed for $(dG-dC)_n$ and $(dI-^5brdC)_n$ in high salt permitting the unambiguous interpretation of a dinucleotide repeat for these synthetic DNA's in high salt solution. The sequence specificity of ligand binding to alternating purine-pyrimidine synthetic DNA's can also be probed by ^{31}P NMR spectroscopy as demonstrated by the observation of resolved resonances corresponding to dTpdA and dApdT phosphodiester linkages in the nitroaniline dication· poly(dA-dT) complexes in solution.

Recent circular dichroism studies have demonstrated that poly(dA-dT) inverts its 260-280 nm spectral bands in high CsF solution [83]. We intend to probe this non-cooperative conformational change by monitoring proton and phosphorous NMR parameters for the synthetic DNA as a function of CsF concentration. Our current attempts are focussed towards the study of fluorine and deuterium labelled nitroaniline dications and steroid diamines in attempts to further characterize the structure and dynamics of ligand-DNA complexes in solution.

Acknowledgment

The nitroaniline dication was synthesized in the laboratory of the late Professor E. Gabbay. We received dipyrandium (synthesized by May and Baker Laboratories, Essex, United Kingdom) from Professor H. Sobell. The correlation NMR spectra of exchangeable protons in H_2O solution were recorded on the Bruker WH-360 at the Mid Atlantic NIH Regional Facility at the University of Pennsylvania Medical School (sponsored by NIH grant RR542).

References

1. E. F. Gale, E. Cunliffe, P. E. Reynolds, M. H. Richmond, and M. J. Waring, *Molecular Basis of Antibiotic Action*, 173-278 (1972).
2. J. Meienenhofer and E. Atherton, in *Structure-Activity Relationships Among the Semi-Synthetic Antibiotics*, Academic Press, New York, 1977, pp. 427-529.
3. E. Gabbay, in *BioOrganic Chemistry III*, (E. E. VanTamelen, ed.), Academic Press, New York, 1977, pp. 33-70.
4. S. Neidle, *Progr. Medicinal Chemistry, 16*:151 (1979).
5. H. M. Sobell, in *International Symposium on Biomolecular Structure, Conformation, Function and Evolution*, (R. Srinivasan, ed.), Pergamon Press, Oxford, 1980.
6. A. Rich, G. J. Quigley and A. H. J. Wang, in *Stereodynamics of Molecular Systems*, (R. H. Sarma, ed.), Pergamon Press, New York, 1979, pp. 315-330.
7. H. M. Berman and S. Neidle, in *Stereodynamics of Molecular Systems*, (R. H. Sarma, ed.), Pergamon Press, New York, 1979 pp. 367-382.
8. N. C. Seeman, in *Nucleic Acid Geometry and Dynamics*, (R. H. Sarma, ed.), Pergamon Press, New York, 1980, pp. 109-142.

9. N. R. Kallenbach and H. M. Berman, *Quarterly Reviews Biophysics, 10*:138 (1977).
10. D. R. Kearns, *Ann. Rev. Biophys. Bioeng., 6*:477 (1977).
11. D. J. Patel, *Acc. Chem. Res., 12*:118 (1979).
12. T. R. Krugh and M. E. Nuss, in *Biological Applications of Magnetic Resonances*, (R. G. Shulman, ed.) Academic Press, New York, 1979, pp. 113-175.
13. D. J. Patel, in *Peptides, Polypeptides and Proteins*, (E. R. Blout, F. A. Bovey, M. Goodman and N. J. Lotan, eds.), Wiley and Sons, New York, 1974, pp. 459-471.
14. D. J. Patel, in *Nucleic Acid Geometry and Dynamics*, (R. H. Sarma, ed.), Pergamon Press, New York, 1980, pp. 185-231.
15. D. J. Patel, in *NMR and ESR of Macromolecules*, (F. A. Bovey and A. Woodward, eds.) American Chemical Society Publications, Washington, D.C., 1980, pp. 219-294.
16. D. J. Patel, L. L. Canuel and F. M. Pohl, *Proc. Natl. Acad. Sci. U.S.A., 76*:2508 (1979).
17. F. M. Pohl and T. M. Jovin, *J. Mol. Biol., 67*:375 (1972).
18. A. H. J. Wang, G. J. Quigley, F. J. Kolpak, J. L. Crawford, J. H. van Boom, G. van der Marel and A. Rich, *Nature, 282*:680 (1979).
19. D. J. Patel, *Eur. J. Biochemistry, 83*:453 (1978).
20. D. R. Kearns, D. J. Patel and R. G. Shulman, *Nature, 229*:338 (1971).
21. C. W. Hilbers, in *Biological Applications of Magnetic Resonance*, (R. G. Shulman, ed.), Academic Press, New York, 1979, pp. 1-44.
22. D. J. Patel, *Biopolymers, 15*:533 (1976).
23. D. J. Patel, *Biopolymers, 16*:1635 (1977).
24. R. L. Baldwin, *Acc. Chem. Res., 4*:265 (1971).
25. R. L. Baldwin, in *Molecular Associations in Biology*, Academic Press, New York, 1968, pp. 145-162.
26. C. Spatz and R. L. Baldwin, *J. Mol. Biol., 11*:213 (1965).
27. C. Giessner-Prettre, B. Pullman, P.N. Borer, L.S. Kan and P. O. P. T'so, *Biopolymers, 15*:2277 (1976).
28. D. B. Arter and P. G. Schmidt, *Nucleic Acids Research, 3*:1427 (1976).
29. E. Palececk, *Progr. Nucleic Acids Research and Molecular Biology, 18*:151 (1976).
30. S. Brahms, J. Brahms and K. E. Van Holde, *Proc. Natl. Acad. Sci. U.S.A., 73*:3453 (1976).
31. M. Levitt, *Proc. Natl. Acad. Sci. U.S.A., 75*:640 (1978).
32. M. Hogan, N. Dattagupta and D. M. Crothers, *Proc. Natl. Acad. Sci. U.S.A., 75*:195 (1978).
33. R. Wing, H. Drew, T. Takano, C. Broka, S. Tanaka, K. Itakura, and R. E. Dickerson, *Nature 287*:755 (1980).
34. D. J. Patel, in *Stereodynamics of Molecular Systems*, (R. H. Sarma, ed.), Pergamon Press, New York, 1979, pp. 397-422.
35. H. Shindo, R. T. Simpson and J. S. Cohen, *J. Biol. Chem., 254*:8125 (1979).

36. F. M. Pohl, *Nature, 260*:365 (1976).
37. C. M. Mercardo and M. Tomasz, *Biochemistry, 16*:2039 (1977).
38. F. M. Pohl, T. M. Jovin, W. Baehr and J. J. Holbrook, *Proc. Natl. Acad. Sci. U.S.A., 69*:3805 (1972).
39. H. R. Drew, R. E. Dickerson and K. Itakura, *J. Mol. Biol., 125*:535 (1978).
40. H. Drew, T. Takano, S. Tanaka, K. Itakura and R. E. Dickerson, *Nature, 286*:567 (1980).
41. J. L. Crawford, F. J. Kolpak, A. H. J. Wang, G. J. Quigley, H. J. van Boom, G. van der Marel, and A. RIch, *Proc. Natl. Acad. Sci. U.S.A., 77*:4016 (1980).
42. S. Arnott, R. Chandrasekaran, B. L. Birdsall, A. G. W. Leslie and R. L. Ratliff, *Nature, 283*:743 (1980).
43. A. Klug, A. Jack, M. A. Viswamitra, O. Kennard, Z. Shakked and T. A. Steitz, *J. Mol. Biol., 131*:669 (1979).
44. M. A. Viswamitra, O. Kennard, P. G. Jones, G. M. Sheldrick, S. Salisbury, L. Falvello, and Z. Shakked, *Nature, 273*: 687 (1978).
45. I. E. Scheffler, E. L. Elson and R. L. Baldwin, *J. Mol. Biol., 36*:291 (1968).
46. P. J. G. Butler and G. P. Lomonossoff, unpublished results (1980).
47. Y. Mitsui, R. Langridge, B. E. Shortle, C. R. Cantor, R. C. Grant, M. Kodama and R. D. Wells, *Nature, 228*:1166 (1970).
48. E. J. Gabbay, *J. Am. Chem. Soc., 91*:5136 (1969).
49. D. J. Patel and C. W. Hilbers, *Biochemistry, 14*:2651 (1975).
50. H. Teitelbaum and S. W. Englander, *J. Mol. Biol., 92*:55, 79 (1975).
51. N. R. Kallenbach, C. Mandel and S. W. Englander, in *Nucleic Acid Geometry and Dynamics*, (R. H. Sarma, ed.), Pergamon Press, New York, 1980, pp. 233-251.
52. C. E. Johnson and F. A. Bovey, *J. Chem. Phys., 29*:1012 (1958).
53. C. Giessner-Prettre and B. Pullman, *J. Theor. Biol., 65*: 171 (1977).
54. H. Shindo and S. B. Zimmerman, *Nature, 76*:2703 (1979).
55. M. S. Barkeley and B. H. Zimm, *J. Chem. Phys., 70*:2991 (1979).
56. P. H. Bolton and T. L. James, *J. Am. Chem. Soc., 102*:25 (1979).
57. T. A. Early and D. R. Kearns, *Proc. Natl. Acad. Sci. U.S.A., 76*:4165 (1979).
58. M. E. Hogan and O. Jardetzky, *Proc. Natl. Acad. Sci. U.S.A., 76*:6341 (1979).
59. W. K. Olson, in *Stereodynamics of Molecular Systems*, (R. H. Sarma, ed.), Pergamon Press, New York, 1979, pp. 297-314.
60. E. D. Lozansky, H. M. Sobell and M. Lessen, in *Stereodynamics of Molecular Systems*, (R. H. Sarma, Pergamon Press, New York, 1979, pp. 265-270.
61. N. R. Kallenbach, C. Mandel and S. W. Englander, in *Stereodynamics of Molecular Systems*, (R. H. Sarma, ed.), Pergamon Press, New York, 1979, pp. 271-282.
62. A. Rich, G. J. Quigley and A. H. J. Wang, in *Nucleic Acid Geometry and Dynamics*, (R. H. Sarma, ed.), Pergamon Press, New York, 1980.
63. F. H. C. Crick and A. Klug, *Nature, 255*:530 (1975).
64. H. M. Sobell, C. C. Tsai, S. G. Gilbert, S. C. Jain and T. D. Sakore, *Proc. Natl. Acad. Sci. U.S.A., 73*:3068 (1976).

65. J. L. Sussman and E. N. Trifonov, *Proc. Natl. Acad. Sci. U.S.A., 75*:103 (1978).
66. M. Levitt, *Proc. Natl. Acad. Sci. U.S.A., 75*:1775 (1978).
67. H. M. Sobell, S. C. Jain, and S. G. Gilbert, *J. Mol. Biol., 114*: 333 (1977).
68. H. R. Mahler, G. Green, R. Goutarel and G. Khuong-Huu, *Biochemistry, 7*:1568 (1968).
69. E. J. Gabbay and R. Glaser, *Biochemistry, 10*:1665 (1971).
70. S. Silver, L. Wendt and P. Bhattacharyya, in *Antibiotics III*, (J. Corcoran and F. E. Hahn, eds.), Springer-Verlag, Heidelberg, 1975, pp. 614-622.
71. M. J. Waring, *J. Mol. Biol., 54*:247 (1970).
72. M. J. Waring and J. W. Chisolm, *Biochem. Biophys. Acta. 262*:18 (1972).
73. M. J. Waring and S. M. Henley, *Nucleic Acids Research, 2*: 567 (1975).
74. J. M. Saucier, *Biochemistry, 16*:5879 (1977).
75. G. Manning, *Biopolymers, 18*:2357 (1979).
76. N. Dattagupta, M. Hogan and D. M. Crothers, *Proc. Natl. Acad. Sci. U.S.A., 75*:4286 (1978).
77. D. J. Patel and L. L. Canuel, *Proc. Natl. Acad. Sci. U.S.A., 76*:24 (1979).
78. R. I. Cotter and D. M. J. Lilley, *FEBS Letters, 82*:63 (1977).
79. N. R. Kallenbach, D. W. Appleby and C. H. Bradley, *Nature 272*:134 (1978).
80. L. Klevan, I. M. Armitage and D. M. Crothers, *Nucleic Acid Research, 6*:1607 (1979).
81. R. T. Simpson and H. Shindo, *Nucleic Acids Research, 7*:481 (1979).
82. R. T. Simpson and H. Shindo, *Nucleic Acids Research, 8*:2093 (1980).
83. M. Varlickova, J. Kypr, V. Kleinwachter and M. Palecek, *Nucleic Acids Research, 8*:3965 (1980).

CHAPTER 6

PROPERTIES OF THE PHOSPHODIESTER BACKBONE OF DUPLEX DNA AND FILAMENTOUS BACTERIOPHAGE DNA

Stanley J. Opella and Joseph A. DiVerdi
Department of Chemistry
University of Pennsylvania
Philadelphia, Pennsylvania

I. INTRODUCTION

The structural and dynamical properties of intact functional biological systems are of greater interest than those of the constituent isolated subunits. However, far less is known about structures with mass greater than 10^6 daltons than those around 10^4 daltons. Much of this discrepancy in knowledge is due to the difficulty of applying diffraction and spectroscopic techniques to very large and complex systems, especially those that cannot be crystallized.

NMR spectroscopy of very large molecules or aggregates is particularly difficult because of the possibilities for overlap or interference among the resonances from the large number of nuclei with similar properties and because of the restrictions on rotational diffusion that accompany large size and the presence of tertiary and quaternary structure. The lack of rapid molecular motions means that the resonances are severely broadened by static nuclear spin interactions, such as dipolar couplings or chemical shift anisotropy, or very efficient nuclear spin relaxation. The combination of many similar resonance signals and broad lines severely limits the technique. While some advantage can be gained from specific isotopic labelling, in general there is little that can be done with proteins that are large by virtue of having many residues in a single polypeptide chain. Those biological systems that are aggregates of small subunits are feasible for study, since the number of overlapping resonances is not overwhelming and the linewidth problem can be directly approached with high resolution solid state NMR techniques. This strategy relies on radiofrequency irradiation or mechanical sample spinning to average out the static linebroadening mechanisms that are present in these samples; experimental methods take the place of rotational diffusion to narrow the lines [1]. The most useful experiments leave one interaction for examination while removing all others.

High molecular weight duplex DNA presents a very difficult magnetic resonance problem in spite of its being a copolymer of only four types of monomers because of its large size and inconvenient motional properties. The integration of solid state and solution NMR techniques is essential for the study of DNA because of its intermediate motional properties. Filamentous bacteriophages are long nucleoprotein rods of 16×10^6 daltons particle weight, where single stranded circular DNA is packaged inside a tube of coat proteins [2]. The highly constrained structure of these viruses means that solid state NMR methods are necessary for their investigation.

II. DOUBLE STRANDED DNA

While the main structural features of DNA are generally regarded as established from diffraction studies of fibers [3,4] as well as oligonucleotide crystals [5], much less is known about the dynamical properties of DNA. The structure of DNA as it is significantly affected by its environment of proteins, drugs, ions, etc. is not well characterized; in these situations more than structural details are of interest, since the motions of DNA are an important influence on conformational flexibility [6,7]. In general, the dynamics of native double stranded DNA have not been described, although processes with rates varying over at least ten orders of magnitude have been detected experimentally [8,9]. Theoretical studies also suggest that a wide range of motions are present in DNA [10].

NMR spectroscopy can, in principal, provide a detailed description of the microscopic dynamics of all atoms in a molecule. However, NMR studies of high molecular weight duplex DNA are problematical because of the very broad linewidths of nucleotide resonances that are a consequence of the motion of the polymer being too slow to effectively average out static nuclear spin linebroadening mechanisms [11]. Therefore, most previous NMR studies of nucleic acids have utilized oligonucleotides [12], single stranded polynucleotides [13], or small fragments of double helical DNA [14-18]. These samples give narrow resonances and can be studied using conventional solution NMR instrumentation and techniques. There have been two preliminary reports of ^{31}P NMR spectra of high molecular weight DNA [19,20].

A. ^{31}P NMR of DNA

The analysis of the phosphorus resonance linewidth from native high molecular weight DNA leads to a description of DNA dynamics [21]. Theoretical and experimental aspects of solid state and solution NMR are required for the study of DNA because the polymer has dynamical characteristics between these two states. The use of ^{31}P NMR obviates any resolution or assignment problems, since the phosphorus nuclei are uniformly located in the phosphodiester backbone of DNA.

The linewidth analysis is carried out by measuring the full width at half maximum height, $\nu_{1/2}$, for the DNA phosphorus resonance as a function of the applied magnetic field strength, B_o, proton decoupling, magic angle sample spinning and temperature. The width of nuclear resonance signals results from the interactions of the nuclear spin with the applied magnetic field and nearby spins. [31]P has nuclear spin of 1/2, therefore dipole-dipole couplings and chemical shift anisotropy are the interactions most likely to affect the linewidth. Dipole-dipole interactions arise from the mutual magnetic coupling through space of two or more nuclei with nonzero spin. In a rigid lattice, the dipolar interactions split the energy levels, resulting in broadening due to the sum of the splittings from the various neighboring nuclei. Chemical shift anisotropy (CSA) arises from the nonspherical distribution of electrons in the phosphate group screening the applied magnetic field to different extents, depending on the orientation of the group in the magnetic field. CSA in solids results in a characteristic chemical shift powder pattern for the line shape of polycrystalline samples [22].

The dipolar and CSA interactions of solid DNA are illustrated with ^{31}P NMR spectra of fibrous DNA in Figure 1. These spectra were obtained by cross-polarization of the phosphorus nuclei from the abundant protons for increased sensitivity [23]. Figure 1A is a broad, nearly featureless resonance that represents the natural ^{31}P lineshape of solid DNA; the approximately 10 kHz linewidth is due to the sum of all [31]P - [31]P and [31]P - [1]H dipolar splittings and the ^{31}P chemical shift anisotropy. The application of strong radiofrequency irradiation at the proton resonance frequency decouples the [31]P - [1]H dipolar interaction giving the characteristic asymmetric chemical shift powder pattern of a phosphodiester in Figure 1B. About 5 kHz of Gaussian linebroadening is removed with proton decoupling, reflecting the magnitude of the [31]P - [1]H dipolar interactions.

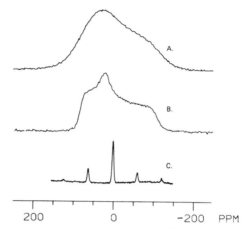

Figure 1. ^{31}P NMR spectra (60.9 MHz) of solid DNA. All spectra are taken using cross-polarization with a 5μ sec 90° pulse, 1 msec mix time, and 1 sec recycle time. (a) stationary powder, 1000 scans, without proton decoupling, (b) as in (a) except with 23 G proton decoupling during acquisition, (c) as in (b) except with magic angle sample spinning at 3.7 kHz.

The principal values of the DNA phosphate chemical shielding tensor can be read off as the discontinuities of the powder spectrum of Figure 1B as $\sigma_{11} = 85$ ppm, $\sigma_{22} = 25$ ppm, and $\sigma_{33} = -109$ ppm relative to external phosphoric acid; these values are within experimental error of those previously reported [24,25]. Rapid rotation of a powder sample at the magic angle ($\Theta = 55°$) with respect to the applied magnetic field averages the chemical shift anisotropy to its isotropic value ($\sigma_{iso} = (\sigma_{11} + \sigma_{22} + \sigma_{33})/3$) [26]. The combination of proton decoupling and magic angle sample spinning gives the ^{31}P spectrum shown in Figure 1C. There is a sharp single line near 0 ppm, the isotropic chemical shift, flanked by spinning sidebands separated by the rotation rate of 3.5 kHz.

The linebroadening from static nuclear spin interactions can be significantly reduced in magnitude by molecular motion. Rapid isotropic motion, as in a liquid, removes the influence of static nuclear interactions and gives to a first approximation an infinitely sharp line when the effective motions are fast compared to the magnitude of the interactions. Linebroadening of motionally averaged resonances can occur through nuclear spin relaxation with the observed linewidth at half-height determined by T_2, the transverse relaxation time according to $\nu_{1/2} = 1/\pi T_2$. Both dipolar couplings and CSA can induce nuclear relaxation, since the asymmetric local fields they generate at the nuclear site are made time dependent by motion. When there is substantial spectral density near the nuclear Larmor, frequency efficient relaxation and linebroadening are induced [27].

DNA in solution is characterized by the ^{31}P NMR spectra in Figure 2. Figure 2B is a spectrum obtained at 61 MHz in a 3.5T field; it has a linewidth of about 800 Hz at 30°C. The reduction of the 10 kHz linewidth from all interactions in Figure 1A to the .8 kHz width of Figure 2B reflects the motional averaging that occurs in solution compared to the rigid lattice. The comparison of Figure 1B and 2C is even more valuable, since proton decoupling was employed and only the chemical shift interaction is influencing the linewidth.

The spectra of DNA in solution shown in Figure 2 illustrate the experiments performed to sort out the contributions to the linewidth. The ^{31}P resonance linewidth measured at 145 MHz (Figure 2A) is much larger than that at 61 MHz (Figure 2B), therefore the linebroadening mechanism has a strong dependence on the strength of the applied magnetic field. The comparison of Spectra 2B and 2C shows that the application of proton decoupling strong enough to remove ^{31}P - ^{1}H dipolar broadening in solids

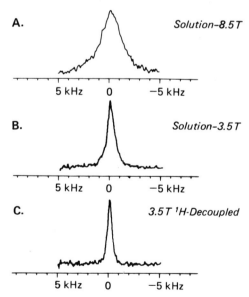

Figure 2. ^{31}P NMR spectra of solution DNA. All spectra are pulsed FID's and 20 mg/ml in high molecular weight DNA. (a) 145 MHz without proton decoupling, (b) 61 MHz without proton decoupling, (c) 61 MHz, 20 G proton decoupling.

narrows the resonance line at 61 MHz by about 400 Hz, therefore a relatively small amount of static dipolar coupling is present in DNA in solution.

Figure 3 shows that the phosphorus resonance linewidth of DNA in solution depends on the square of the applied magnetic field strength. This dependence is completely diagnostic for chemical shift anisotropy relaxation as the linebroadening mechanism [27]. If the entire DNA phosphate linewidth is due to CSA relaxation, then the plot of linewidth versus field strength squared should pass through the origin; instead the intercept at zero field is about 400 Hz.

The proton decoupling experiment in Figures 2B and 2C shows that 400 Hz of broadening is due to ^{31}P - ^{1}H couplings. This can account for the 400 Hz intercept, since the strength of dipole-dipole interactions are independent of applied magnetic field strength. By subtracting the dipolar part from the total observed linewidth, the solid line plot of Figure 3 is generated; this line now has the squared field dependence and zero intercept of CSA relaxation.

There are two spin interactions that dominate the ^{31}P resonance linewidth of DNA in solution: CSA relaxation and ^{31}P - ^{1}H static dipolar couplings. The combination of magnetic field strength dependence and decoupling experiments separates these two effects. There are probably

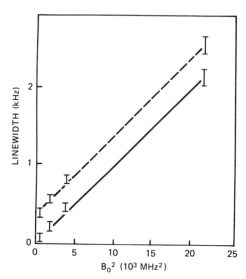

Figure 3. Magnetic field strength dependence of ^{31}P linewidth in solution DNA. Dashed line is without proton decoupling, solid line is proton decoupled.

additional interactions that make relatively small contributions to the phosphorus resonance linewidth that are not apparent in this analysis because of errors in measurement of linewidth and temperature, as well as because their influence is simply overwhelmed by the two large effects; the most likely candidates are dispersion of the isotropic chemical shift among the various phosphates (.5 ppm) and heteronuclear dipolar relaxation.

B. Dynamics of Duplex DNA

The phosphodiester linkage of DNA in solution has substantial mobility. This is the reason for the drastic linewidth for DNA in solution compared to the rigid solid for all spin interactions (Figures 1A and 2B) as well as just the chemical shift (Figures 1B and 2C). Three different nuclear spin interactions influence the linewidth of the phosphorus resonance of DNA in solution with three different timescales. The motional averaging reduces static chemical shift anisotropy and static ^{31}P - ^{1}H dipolar couplings, and induces nuclear spin relaxation due to the fluctuating fields generated by the chemical shift anisotropy.

Quantitative interpretation of these parameters gives a description of the motions of DNA in solution. The motion of the phosphodiester backbone of DNA is fast enough to completely average the 10^4 Hz static phosphorus chemical shift anisotropy, although it does not fully average the 5×10^3 Hz static ^{31}P - ^{1}H dipolar broadening. This discrepancy in frequency scales can be explained in several ways. First of all, the chemical shift powder pattern is a "tent-like" shape with abrupt discontinuities at the frequency limits of σ_{11} and σ_{33} (10 kHz at 61 MHz), while the dipolar ^{31}P - ^{1} broadening has the form of a Gaussian function with some intensity significantly beyond the nominal 5×10^3 Hz at half height of the static interaction. Therefore, more rapid motions are required to completely remove the broadening from the dipolar couplings than the equivalent chemical shift anisotropy. The same argument is used in describing the formation of spinning sidebands separate from the centerband at rotation rates on the order of or less than the magnitude of the chemical shift anisotropy [28]; and this is illustrated in Figure 1C where rotation at 3.5×10^3 Hz is sufficient to transform the 10×10^3 Hz chemical shift powder pattern to a recognizable isotropic chemical shift line with small sidebands. Another reason may be that the effective motion is not isotropic and the chemical shielding and dipolar tensors respond differently to rotations along various molecular axes.

Rates of rotational diffusion can be determined from nuclear magnetic resonance relaxation parameters, such as linewidth, when the relaxation mechanism is known. Figure 3 gives the linewidth of DNA phosphates due only to chemical shift anisotropy relaxation. In principle, a thorough relaxation analysis including longitudinal and transverse relaxation processes that utilizes the complete chemical shielding tensor of the phosphodiester group could characterize the rates and directions of the group on DNA in solution. The more limited data set of the principal values of the chemical shielding tensor combined with the CSA relaxation induced linewidth can give a rotational diffusion constant for the phosphate group that is explicitly restricted to isotropic reorientation. At 30°C the observed linewidth at 145 MHz is 2.15 kHz of which 400 Hz is due to ^{31}P - ^{1}H dipolar interactions, so the linewidth due to CSA relaxation is 1.75 kHz which corresponds to an isotropic rotational correlation time of about 2×10^{-6} sec for the phosphodiester group of DNA. This value can only be considered an order of magnitude estimate because of the assumption that the motion is isotropic.

However, all of the NMR results are consistent with the phosphodiester motions of DNA being isotropic. If rotations in one or a few directions were rapid while other motions were slow, then axially symmetric chemical shift powder patterns reduced in magnitude would result for the phosphorus resonances; this does not occur for DNA in solution and indicates that rotations in all directions are fast compared to 10^4 Hz. The rotational diffusion constant, $D_{rot} = 1/6\tau_c = 8 \times 10^4 sec^{-1}$, where τ_c is the rotational correlation time calculated above at 30°C. This rate is greater than the 10^4 Hz static CSA and the 5×10^3 Hz static dipolar couplings, but not so much larger that it is unreasonable that some portion ($\sim 10\%$) of the residual dipolar broadening is unaveraged by the motion.

The phosphate groups of DNA undergo rotational diffusion at a substantial rate. High molecular weight native DNA is a flexible polymer rather than a rigid rod. The primary question we wish to address in the interpretation of DNA dynamics, is whether the phosphate motions are consistent with the relatively long range flexibility of the polymer or if there are local motions of the backbone.

Hydrodynamic results show that DNA has a persistence length of about 180 base pairs [29]. This corresponds to the distance on the chain between independently oriented nucleotides. Bending motions occur in all directions giving rise to essentially isotropic motion at a given position in the chain. A correlation time resulting from long range bending of DNA can be calculated to be between 10^{-7} and 10^{-5} sec [10,30]. The rotational correlation time determined from these ^{31}P NMR results is near 10^{-6} sec. If the flexibility of the polymer due to bending motions corresponds to rotational rates around 10^{-6}sec, then there is no evidence for internal phosphate motions in high molecular weight native DNA and the phosphodiester group motions correspond to the bending motions.

III. FILAMENTOUS DNA PHAGES

The filamentous bacteriophages are long thin rods of DNA and protein. There are a number of related viruses in this category with somewhat different structures. fd from infected Escherichia coli and Pf1 from Pseudomonas aeruginosa represent the extremes of overall length with fd being 0.9μ long and Pf1 2μ long even though the number of nucleotides in their DNAs is similar (6400 vs 7400). Comparitive studies of their DNA offer some advantages for interpretation and understanding the possibilities for packing arrangements of DNA-protein complexes [31,32].

There is a substantial amount of experimental evidence that filamentous bacteriophages have their DNA extended lengthwise within a tubular chamber made from the major coat protein subunits [35]. Simple design principles are expected for biological supramolecular structures like viruses, yet there are significant problems outstanding in the description of filamentous viruses especially with regard to how the DNA is packed inside the coat protein shell. X-ray diffraction data combined with molecular model building have shown that the coat proteins are arranged in an overlapping helical array. While the details of the coat protein helix are under active investigation there is little doubt that the protein shell of these viruses is highly symmetrical [34,35]. In contrast, there is little known about the arrangement of the DNA in the virus interior or the interactions between the DNA and the proteins.

The difficulties with understanding the architecture of the filamentous phages as nucleoprotein complexes start at the most basic level. After all, it is not obvious why a circular DNA is packaged in a long cylinder, especially when there is no evidence for basepairing in the DNA. The X-ray diffraction results that have been interpreted to give the models for the coat protein shell do not have intensity recognizable as from the DNA [36,37]. Therefore, there is no diffraction data on how the DNA is arranged or how the nucleotides interact with the amino acids of the coat protein. A particularly important difference between fd and Pf1 is their ratio of nucleotides to coat proteins which is 2.3 for fd and 1.0 for Pf1 [31]. The noninteger ratio for fd is difficult to reconcile with most plausible models of symmetrical DNA-protein interactions, while the drastic difference between these two ratios is in contrast to the strong similarities between these viruses in other respects.

One of the goals of the NMR studies of these viruses is to describe the structure and the packing of their DNA [35]. There are few other spectroscopic means of separating the nucleotide and aromatic amino acid chromophores. Day and coworkers have had to rely almost exclusively on physico-chemical characterization of the virus particles to propose models for the DNA arrangements [31,32]. Photochemical crosslinking experiments indicate that a small part of fd DNA exists in a hairpin structure and this may fix the location of the DNA relative to one end of the particle, although this approach gives no indication of overall packing arrangements of the DNA [39].

A. Structural Properties From ^{31}P NMR

NMR spectroscopy of the coat proteins and DNA of these viruses can contribute to understanding their structure, dynamics and assembly [38,40-45]. Since the only phosphorus atoms in these viruses are in the phosphodiester linkages of the DNA backbone, ^{31}P NMR gives information on the DNA without interference from the more abundant coat proteins [44]. Structural properties of the viral DNA can be obtained from the ^{31}P chemical shift parameters, ^{31}P - ^{31}P dipolar couplings, and ^{31}P -^{1}H dipolar couplings. Dynamical properties of the DNA for the viruses in solution is available from the motional averaging of these spin interactions.

The chemical shielding properties of the phosphates of fd in the solid state are characterized by the spectra in Figure 4. These spectra were obtained with high-power proton decoupling to remove ^{31}P - ^{1}H dipolar interactions. Spectrum 4A is of a stationary sample of solid fd; it is the chemical shift powder pattern of the phosphates. The breadth and shape are from the asymmetric phosphodiester chemical shielding tensor with a small amount of broadening due to ^{31}P - ^{31}P dipolar couplings. The principal values of the fd phosphorus chemical shielding tensor can be determined directly from the discontinuities of Spectrum 4A as $\sigma_{11} = 85$ ppm, $\sigma_{22} = 22$ ppm and $\sigma_{33} = -109$ ppm. The spectra of Figure 4 are from lyophilized samples of fd, however the spectrum of Figure 4A is indistinguishable from that obtained from a frozen solution of fd. The powder spectrum of Pf1 differs slightly from fd in the shape and intensity only near σ_{33}.

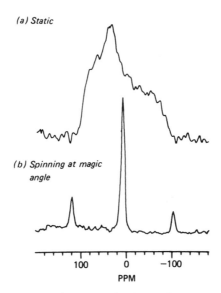

^{31}P NMR OF fd VIRUS

(a) Static

(b) Spinning at magic angle

100   0   −100

PPM

Figure 4. ^{31}P NMR spectra (60.9 MHz) of solid fd. Both spectra were obtained using cross-polarization with the same parameter as in Figure 1 with 23 G proton decoupling. (a) stationary powder, 10,000 scans, (b) as in (a) except with magic angle sample spinning at 4.5 kHz.

The spectrum of Figure 4B was obtained on the same sample used in Figure 4A, except that it was placed in an Andrew Beams rotor and spun at 4.5 kHz at the magic angle ($\Theta = 55°$) with respect to the applied magnetic field. The magic angle spinning averages out the ^{31}P CSA to give the isotropic chemical shift spectrum as a single line at -0.9 ppm. Since the magic angle spinning spectrum has only a single centerband, the powder spectrum is representative of one type of phosphate. The principal elements and isotropic chemical shift of this phosphate are the same within experimental error, of those observed in Figure 1 for calf thymus DNA or isolated fd DNA. The ^{31}P chemical shift parameters are not altered by packaging within the coat protein shell of the virion; there is no evidence of distortion of the DNA backbone or otherwise altered chemical structures.

The dipole-dipole interaction is well suited for molecular structure determinations because of its simple dependence on distance and angles [46]. While angular information can only be obtained from oriented samples, distance information is accessible in polycrystalline or amorphous samples. Since the strength of the dipolar couplings falls off rapidly with distance it is sensitive to nearest neighbors which simplifies many of the calculations.

The dipolar coupling between ^{31}P nuclei can be used to obtain structure parameters of biological structures. Experimentally, ^{31}P - ^{31}P dipolar couplings can be arranged to be the dominant spin interaction by decoupling the ^{31}P - ^{31}H dipolar interactions with radiofrequency irradiation and applying pulses to cancel out the ^{31}P chemical shift effects. The ^{31}P - ^{31}P homonuclear dipolar interactions in powder samples is most conveniently expressed in terms of a second moment as in the well known Van Vleck [47] formula

$$M_2 = 9/20(h\gamma_p^2)^2 \sum_{j>k} r^{-6}_{jk}$$

Where M_2 is the phosphous second moment, γ_p is the phosphorus gyromagnetic ratio, and r_{jk} is the distance between the jth and k^{th} phosphorus.

The actual experiment performed on the phosphorus resonance consists of developing ^{31}P magnetization along the X axis of a rotating reference frame and forming a spin-echo with a 180° pulse at the phosphorus frequency under proton decoupling. The loss of signal intensity as a function of time of echo formation, τ reflects the strength of the ^{31}P - ^{31}P dipolar couplings. Since dipolar broadening takes the form of convolution of the frequency domain with a Gaussian, the time domain signal will also drop off as a Gaussian function. This is described by equation (2).

$$I_p(\tau) = I_p(o) \exp(-2\pi^2 M_2\tau^2)$$

where $I_p(\tau)$ is the integrated intensity at time $= \tau$

Figure 5 shows the plots of Pf1 and fd phosphorus intensity as a function of time for this procedure. The log of the observed intensity falls off as τ^2. In these rigid solid samples the ^{31}P - ^{31}P couplings reflect structure.

The phosphate-phosphate distances, on average, are different for fd and Pf1 according to Figure 5. The single parameter of phosphorus second moment reflects averages over several constants, therefore interpretation at this stage must rely on independent evidence and fitting proposed models. The DNA in both viruses is a circle of single stranded DNA. It is confined within a cylindrical core region of about 20 Å in diameter as deduced from X-ray diffraction data. Mechanical shearing experiments

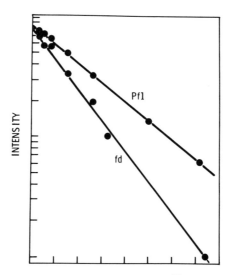

Figure 5. Plot of integral of observed intensity of ^{31}P resonance (60.9 MHz) vs time squared of evolution under phosphorus-phosphorus dipole interaction. From the slope of these lines the second moment of this interaction and then a weighted average of phosphorus-phosphorus distances can be obtained.

show that the DNA occupies the entire length of the virus particle so that there exist two antiparallel chains of DNA stretched between the ends of the filament interior. The DNA strands are assumed to be regular helices as shown in the diagram of Figure 6 [32]. However, basepairing does not occur in either fd or Pfl, since the A-T and G-C ratios are not integers. The number of nucleotides for each virus is known as are their total lengths, thus the axial rise per base (projected on the long axis of the virion) can be calculated by dividing the total length of the virus particle by 1/2 the number of bases. The axial rise per base is 2.8 Å and 5.4 Å for fd and Pfl, respectively.

The DNA helical parameters can be deduced by comparison with coat protein helix parameters. For Pfl there is a one to one stoichiometry between nucleotides and coat protein subunits, and there are 5.4 protein subunits per turn of protein helix. If the bases interact alternately on the up and down chains of the DNA, there are 2.7 bases per turn of DNA helix for each chain giving a twist of the helix per base of 133D [32]. The nonstoichiometric relationship of nucleotides to coat proteins in fd makes the determination of this parameter less certain, but it appears to be between 60° and 72° per base.

(a)   (b)

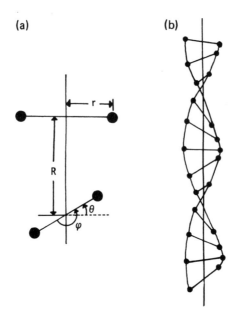

Figure 6. Schematic diagram of the model used for the phosphodiester backbone of DNA packaged in filamentous phages. The right side depicts the general helix structure. Note that base pairing is not implied by the interstrand lines. The left side shows the 4 parameters used to define the helix.

It is assumed that intermolecular repulsions will cause the DNA strands to be maximally distant, i.e., 180° apart looking down the twist axis. It is also assumed that the bases of antiparallel chains are not staggered [32]. This leaves the radial distance of each strand undefined. The second moment of the phosphate resonance was calculated for the five nearest neighbors of any phosphate as a function of the radius of the DNA helix in the virus. For Pf1, the observed second moment corresponds to a radial distance of 4.9 Å, while for fd a range based on the range of helix twist of the bases is 5.4 - 4.8 Å. These data are listed in Table I. It appears, at least to the present level of resolution in the experiment, that the phosphates of fd and Pf1 are located at the same radial distance, midway out of the central cylindrical core. The predominant difference in the packaging of fd and Pf1 DNA appears to be related to the lengthwise stretch in the cylinder rather than radial displacement.

TABLE I

		Pf1	*fd*
$<\Delta\omega^2>$	Hz^2	4.4×10^3	7.3×10^3
R	Å	5.4	2.8
r	Å	4.9	5.4 - 4.8
$\Theta°$		133	60 - 72
$\phi°$		180	180

B. Dynamical Properties From ^{31}P NMR

Molecular motions are reflected in the chemical shielding properties of a site. For a phosphodiester with a total shift anisotropy of 200 ppm at 61 MHz motions faster than about 10^4sec^{-1} will reduce the magnitude of the chemical shift anisotropy while those between about 10^6 and 10^9sec^{-1} will result in efficient nuclear relaxation due to fluctuating fields induced by asymmetric electronic shielding.

The ^{31}P NMR spectrm of solid fd in Figure 7A displays the full chemical shift anisotropy of a phosphodiester group, therefore motions faster than 10^4sec^{-1} are absent in lyophilized powders or frozen solutions of the virus. The influence of water on fd is shown in Figures 7B-7D. These are proton decoupled spectra, therefore only the chemical shift properties are being monitored. Figure 7B is for fd equilibrated in an atmosphere of 92% relative humidity and the principal values of the phosphorus chemical shielding tensor (σ_{11} = 78 ppm, σ_{22} = 16 ppm, σ_{33} = -96 ppm) are somewhat reduced from the values for the completely dehydrated virus. This sample corresponds to the state of fd in the fibers used in the X-ray diffraction experiments. The finding of a large anisotropy for the phosphate shielding rules out molecular motion as an explanation for the lack of diffraction intensity attributable to DNA in the X-ray diffraction patterns. The DNA is clearly not moving independently of the coat protein shell and the backbone does not have rapid local motions.

The spectrum from fd in solution is in Figure 7C. This resonance is broad with slight asymmetry and does not change with the application of proton decoupling. The width near the base of the peak is nearly 200 ppm while the measured width at half height is around 110 ppm (6.5 kHz at 61

³¹P NMR of fd

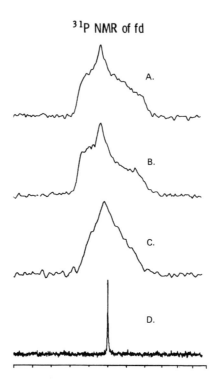

Figure 7. ³¹P NMR (60.9 MHz) of fd DNA. (a), (b) and (c) were taken using cross-polarization with the same parameters as Figure 1 and with 23 G proton decoupling. (d) was taken with a 5μ sec 90° pulse and 10 W proton decoupling. (a) fd powder, 10,000 scans, (b) fd powder, 92% R. H., 10,000 scans, (c) fd solution (50 mg/ml) 50,000 scans and (d) isolated fd DNA in solution, 2000 FID's.

MHz). Even though at first glance the ³¹P resonance of fd and ds DNA may be similar in that they are very broad and not Lorentzian, the detailed analysis shows them to be quite different in origin. The ³¹P resonance linewidth of fd in solution is due to static chemical shift anisotropy that is not averaged by motion. This is demonstrated with several NMR experiments. Figure 8 compares the ³¹P spectra of fd in solution when stationary and when spinning at the magic angle. The moderate rotation rate employed for the spinning breaks up the broad peak into discrete side-bands, therefore the broadening is due to the inhomogeneous chemical shift anisotropy.

The plot of linewidth versus applied magnetic field strength for the fd phosphorus line in Figure 9 shows that the width at half height increases

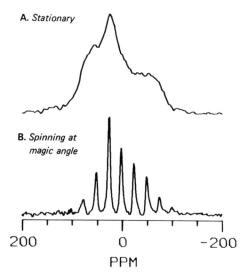

Figure 8. ^{31})P NMR (60.9 MHz) of fd in solution. Both spectra were obtained using cross-polarization using the parameters in Figure 1 and 25 G proton decoupling. (a) stationary fd solution (200 mg/ml), and (b) same as (a) except with magic angle spinning at 2.1 kHz.

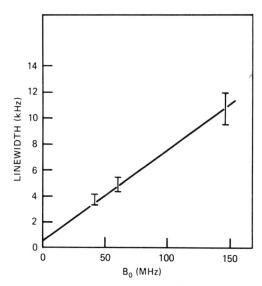

Figure 9. Magnetic field strength dependence of ^{31}P linewidth in fd solution. All spectra were pulsed FID's without proton decoupling.

linearly with field strength. This is the behavior expected for the chemical shift anisotropy powder pattern, but not chemical shift anisotropy relaxation which has a squared field dependence as seen for ds DNA in Figure 3. The rounding of the powder pattern for fd in solution reflects the rotational diffusion of the entire particle [44], therefore there does not appear to be internal phosphate motions present.

Figure 7D is the ^{31}P NMR spectrum of single stranded fd DNA. Like other samples of single stranded DNA [13], the narrow line reflects the presence of rapid backbone motions that average out the static CSA and dipolar interactions. These motions occur on the nanosecond timescale. The comparison of Figure 7C and 7D illustrates the influence of the coat protein on dynamics. fd DNA in solution has rotations with correlation times around 10^{-9}sec and the DNA in the virion has limited amounts of motion faster than 10^{-4}sec.

IV. DNA COMPARISONS

Properties of DNA in three different situations are described by ^{31}P NMR; these are high molecular weight double helical DNA, single stranded DNA, and the DNA of the filamentous viruses. The amount of structural information based on the principal elements of the chemical shielding tensor as the isotropic chemical shifts is disappointing, since these three different DNAs have essentially identical chemical shift properties. Either the ^{31}P chemical shielding is insensitive to the packaging of DNA or these DNAs have very similar backbone conformations and chemistry. The ^{31}P - ^{31}P dipolar couplings can be used to extract structural information for the filamentous viruses, however, this method is of little use for naked DNA where phosphate distances to other helices are less than those on one strand or between strands of one pair. The coat protein shell of the viruses serves to isolate the DNA from other DNA molecules. While the dipolar analysis is at an early stage, it clearly has the potential for describing packing of DNA in nucleoprotein complexes.

A very wide range of motions are observed for DNA, depending on its biological role. Single stranded DNA has very fast backbone reorientations with rates near 10^{-9}sec. Double stranded DNA appears to have no local backbone motions, but since DNA is a flexible polymer the phosphates have a rotational correlation time around 10^{-6}sec. The single stranded DNA of the filamentous viruses is completely immobilized by the protein coat with no evidence of internal rotations or bending motions; only the rotational diffusion of the virus particles about the long axis is apparent.

Acknowledgments

We thank P. Tsang for help preparing the Pfl samples, T. A. Cross for help preparing the fd samples, and W. B. Wise for help with the ^{31}P NMR measurements. The research was supported by the American Cancer Society (NP-225), NIH (GM-24266), and NSF (PCM-05598). S. J. O. is a fellow of the A. P. Sloan Foundation (1980-1982).

References

1. U. Haeberlen and J. S. Waugh, *Phys. Rev., 185*:420 (1969).
2. D. A. Marvin and B. Hohn, *Bacterial Rev., 33*:172 (1969).
3. J. D. Watson and F. H. C. Crick, *Nature, 171*:737 (1953).
4. S. Arnott, *Progr. Biophys. Mol. Biol., 21*:267 (1979).
5. N. R. Kallenbach and H. M. Berman, *Quart. Rev. Biophys., 10*:137 (1977).
6. F. H. C. Crick and A. Klug, *Nature, 255*:530 (1975).
7. H. M. Sobell, C. C. Tsai, S. G. Gilbert, S. C. Jain, and T. D. Sakare, *Proc. Natl. Acad. Sci. U.S., 73*:3068 (1976).
8. P. Wahl, J. Paoletti, and J-B LePecq, *Proc. Natl. Acad. Sci. U.S., 65*:417 (1970).
9. H. Teitelbaum and S. W. Englander, *J. Mol. Biol., 92*:55 (1975).
10. M. D. Barkley and B. H. Zimm, *J. Chem. Phys., 70*:2991 (1979).
11. C. C. McDonald, W. D. Phillips, and S. Penman, *Science, 144*:1234 (1964).
12. P. Davanloo, I. M. Armitage, and D. M. Crothers, *Biopolymers, 18*:663 (1979).
13. K. Akasaka, A. Yamada, and H. Hatano, *Bull. Chem. Soc. Japan, 50*:2858 (1977).
14. T. A. Early and D. R. Kearns, *Proc. Natl. Acad. Sci. U.S., 76*:4165 (1979).
15. M. E. Hogan and O. Jardetzky, *Proc. Natl. Acad. Sci. U.S., 76*:6341 (1979).
16. P. H. Bolton and T. L. James, *J. Am. Chem. Soc., 102*:25 (1980).
17. R. L. Rill, P. R. Hilliard, J. T. Bailey, and G. C. Levy, *J. Am. Chem. Soc., 102*:418 (1980).
18. P. H. Bolton and T. L. James, *Biochemistry, 19*:1388 (1980).
19. S. Hanlon, T. Glonek, and A. Chan, *Biochemistry, 15*:3869 (1976).
20. A. Yamada, H. Kaneko, K. Akasaka, and H. Hatano, *FEBS Lett., 93*:16 (1978).
21. S. J. Opella, W. B. Wise, and J. A. DiVerdi, *Biochemistry, 20*:284 (1981).
22. M. Mehring, *High Resolution NMR Spectroscopy in Solids*, Springer-Verlag, Berlin, 1976.
23. A. Pines, M. G. Gibby, and J. S. Waugh, *J. Chem. Phys., 59*:569 (1973).
24. T. Terao, S. Matsui, and K. Akasaka, *J. Amer. Chem. Soc., 99*:6136 (1977).
25. H. Shindo, J. B. Wooten, B. H. Pheiffer, and S. B. Zimmerman, *Biochemistry, 19*:518 (1980).

26. E. R. Andrew, A. Bradbury, and R. G. Eades, *Nature, 182*:1659 (1958).
27. A. Abragam, *The Principles of Nuclear Magnetism*, Oxford, 1961.
28. J. S. Waugh, M. M. Maricq, and R. Cantor, *J. Mag. Res., 29*:183 (1978).
29. V. A. Bloomfield, D. M. Crothers, and I. Tinoco, *Physical Chemistry of Nucleic Acids*, Harper and Row, N.Y., 1974.
30. P. H. Bolton and T. L. James, *J. Phys. Chem., 83*:3359 (1979).
31. L. A. Day and R. L. Wiseman, *The Single Stranded DNA Phages*, Cold Spring Harbor, N.Y., 1978.
32. L. A. Day, R. L. W. Wiseman, and C. J. Mareic, *Nucleic Acids Res., 7*:1393 (1979).
33. D. A. Marvin and E. J. Wachtel, *Nature, 253*:19 (1975).
34. D. A. Marvin, in *The Single Stranded DNA Phages*, Cold Spring Harbor, N.Y., 1978.
35. L. Makowski and D. L. D. Caspar, *The Single Stranded DNA Phages*, Cold Spring Harbor, N.Y. 1978.
36. D. A. Marvin, R. L. Wiseman, and E. J. Wachtel, *J. Mol. Biol., 82*:121 (1974).
37. D. A. Marvin, W. J. Pigram, R. L. Wiseman, E. J. Wachtel, and F. J. Marvin, *J. Mol. Biol., 88*:581 (1974).
38. T. A. Cross, J. A. DiVerdi, W. B. Wise, and S. J. Opella, in *NMR and Biochemistry* (S. J. Opella and P. Lu, eds.), Kekker, N.Y.:67 1979.
39. C-K Shen, A. Ikoku, and J. E. Hearst, *J. Mol. Biol., 127*:163 (1979).
40. T. A. Cross and S. J. Opella, *J. Supramol. Struct., 11*:139 (1979).
41. S. J. Opella, M. H. Frey, and T. A. Cross, *J. Amer. Chem. Soc., 101*:5856 (1979).
42. T. A. Cross and S. J. Opella, *Biochem. Biophys. Res. Comm., 92*:478 (1980).
43. S. J. Opella, T. A. Cross, J. A. DiVerdi, and C. F. Sturm, *Biophys. J., 32*:531 (1980).
44. J. A. DiVerdi and S. J. Opella, *Biochemistry, 20*:280 (1981).
45. T. A. Cross and S. J. Opella, *Biochemistry, 20*:290 (1981).
46. G. E. Pake, *J. Chem. Phys., 16*:327 (1948).
47. J. H. Van Vleck, *Phys. Rev., 74*:1168 (1948).

CHAPTER 7

THE ELUCIDATION OF THE PRINCIPAL AXIS SYSTEM OF THE MAGNETIC SUSCEPTIBILITY TENSOR OF Yb^{+3} IN THE EF SITE OF CARP PARVALBUMIN AS THE CENTRAL ELEMENT REQUIRED IN THE USE OF LANTHANIDE INDUCED NMR SHIFTS FOR THE DETERMINATION OF PROTEIN STRUCTURE IN SOLUTION.

Lana Lee and Brian D. Sykes
Department of Biochemistry and
MRC Group on Protein Structure and Function
University of Alberta
Edmonton, Alberta
Canada

I. INTRODUCTION

Calcium binding proteins play an important role in the regulation of many biochemical processes [1,2]. Among the most studied of these proteins are the skeletal and cardiac troponins [3], and myosin light chains [4], which are involved in the regulation of muscle contraction; and calmodulin [5] from brain which is involved in the regulation of cyclic nucleotide phosphodiesterase activity. The elucidation of the X-ray structure of the calcium binding protein parvalbumin from carp revealed that each of its two calcium binding sites is completely formed from a contiguous polypeptide sequence folded into the homologous "CD and EF hands" [6]. Each calcium binding site contains two turns of helix, a 12 residue loop around the metal ion, and a second two turn helix. The loop around the metal ion contains regularly spaced liganding carboxyl, hydroxyl, and carbonyl ligands. Homologous sequences to parvalbumin [1,7-9] can be found in many other calcium binding proteins such as those listed above. The number of times in a given protein the sequence repeats, and the substitutions therein, can be correlated with the number of metals bound to the protein and their binding strengths, respectively. These findings have lead to the proposal that homologous structures, at least at the level of the calcium binding sites, exist for all these proteins.

In a separate paper [10] we have discussed the development and strategies of a NMR methodology which will enable us to test this structural hypothesis in solution. The technique is based upon the substitution of a paramagnetic lanthanide ion for the calcium ion, and the subsequent analysis in structural terms of the shifts and broadenings induced in the ^{1}H NMR spectrum of the protein. We have presented the details of the analysis of the broadening of the lanthanide shifted resonances in terms of the distance between the lanthanide metal ion and the shifted nucleus [11]. However, the lanthanide induced shifts are the most sensitive monitors of the precise geometrical orientation of each proton nucleus relative to the metal. The values of several parameters in the equation relating the NMR shifts to the structure are, however, unknown a priori. By studying the lanthanide induced shifts for the protein carp parvalbumin (pI = 4.25), whose structure has been determined by X-ray crystallographic techniques [6], we have attempted to determine these parameters, which are the orientation and principal elements of the magnetic susceptibility tensor of the protein bound lanthanide metal. With these parameters, and the knowledge of the amino acid substitutions for different proteins, we will then be able to compare the calculated and observed NMR spectra of a new protein as a probe of its structure.

The interaction of the lanthanide ytterbium with parvalbumin results in high resolution NMR spectra exhibiting a series of resonances with shifts spread over the range 32 to -19 ppm. The orientation and principal elements of the magnetic susceptibility tensor of ytterbium bound in the EF calcium binding site of parvalbumin have been determined using three assigned NMR resonances, the His-26 C2 and C4 protons and the amino terminal acetyl protons, and seven methyl groups; all with known geometry relative to the EF calcium binding site. The details of the assignment and the measurement of the Yb^{+3} induced shifts for the His-26 C2 and C4 protons and the amino terminal acetyl protons are discussed in detail herein. Also presented is the determination of the Yb^{+3} induced shift of the fluorine resonance of a chemically modified parvalbumin, 2-mercuri-4-fluorophenol-parvalbumin, which was used as a check on the determination of the principal axis system.

The elucidation of the orientation and principal elements of the Yb^{+3} magnetic susceptibility tensor when bound to parvalbumin has allowed us at this stage to compare the observed spectrum of the nuclei surrounding the EF calcium binding site of parvalbumin with that calculated from the X-ray structure. A significant number of the calculated shifts are larger than any of the observed shifts. We feel that a refinement of the X-ray based proton coordinates will be possible utilizing the geometric information contained in the lanthanide shifted NMR spectrum.

II. THEORY OF THE LANTHANIDE INDUCED SHIFTS

When a paramagnetic lanthanide ion (excluding the isotropic Gd^{+3}) is substituted for one or both of the calcium ions of parvalbumin, a series of shifted resonances appear in the ^1H NMR spectrum far outside of the envelope of the spectrum of the calcium form of the protein. The shifted peaks in these spectra, shown in Figure 1 for Yb^{+3} substituted in the EF calcium binding site, are in the NMR slow exchange limit because the inverse of the lifetime of the Yb^{+3} parvalbumin complex is smaller than any of the lanthanide induced shifts for the observed resonances. The

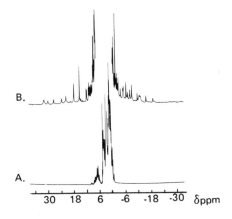

Figure 1. The 270 MHz ^1H NMR spectrum of carp parvalbumin:
A. 0.68 mM calcium saturated carp parvalbumin in 15 mM Pipes, 0.15 M KCl, 0.5 mM DSS, 10 mM DTT, in D_2O, pH 6.65, temperature = 303°K.
B. 0.64 mM carp parvalbumin in 15 mM Pipes, 0.15 M KCl, 0.5 mM DSS, 10 mM DTT in D_2O, pH=6.6, temperature = 303°K, at a total Yb^{+3} to total protein ratio (Yb/P) of 0.80. The vertical scale for Figure b is 8X that of Figure a. The proton chemical shifts are measured with respect to the major resonance of DSS. (From Ref. 10.)

shifted resonances therefore represent the spectrum of the protein-paramagnetic metal ion complex. The shifts result from the influence of the 4f electrons of the lanthanide metal on nearby ^1H nuclei and can be divided into two contributions. The first is a through space dipolar ("pseudo-contact") interaction. The magnitude of the pseudo-contact shift is a function of the metal ion involved and of the geometry of the proton relative to the metal ion. The shift of the nucleus from its diamagnetic position written in the principal axis system of the magnetic susceptibility tensor of the metal ion is [12]

$$\delta_p = A_1 \frac{3\cos^2\theta - 1}{r^3} + A_2 \frac{\sin^2\theta \cos 2\phi}{r^3} \equiv A_1G_1 + A_2G_2$$

where $\mathring{A}_1$ and $\mathring{A}_2$ are parameters related to the principal elements of the magnetic susceptibility tensor of the metal ion, θ, ϕ, and r are the spherical coordinates of the nucleus in the principal axis system, and the { } brackets indicate that the appropriate time averaged geometry of the nucleus must be used in the calculation [13]. With order of magnitude values of $A_1 \approx A_2 \approx 1600$ ppm $\mathring{A}^{+3}$ from other experiments [14], we see that nuclei in the range of $\approx 4\mathring{A}$ from the metal can have shifts as large as ≈ 50 ppm whereas nuclei $\approx 10\mathring{A}$ from the metal can have shifts only as large as ≈ 3 ppm.

The second contribution to the shifts is a through bond contact interaction which we will assume is negligible. This contribution is important for directly bonded nuclei such as ^{13}C and ^{17}O, whereas we are looking at ^1H nuclei several bonds removed. Also it is generally less important for the lanthanides when compared with, for example, the transition metals. We attempt further to minimize this contribution by choice of metal since the geometric dependence of this contribution to the shift is not known a priori. We have chosen Yb^{+3} because the ratio of the pseudo-contact shift to the contact shift is largest, and the absolute value of the contact shift is the smallest, for Yb^{+3} when compared to the other lanthanides [15]. Other criteria are discussed elsewhere [10,11,16].

For the first stage of the development of our NMR methodology, we are interested in the determination of the orientation in the protein of the principal axis system of the magnetic susceptibility tensor of the Yb^{+3}, and the two parameters $\mathring{A}_1 = (X_{zz} - \bar{X}$ and $\mathring{A}_2 = (X_{xx} - X_{yy})$ where X_{xx}, X_{yy}, X_{zz} and $\bar{X}$ are the principal elements and trace respectively of the magnetic susceptibility tensor. (We will assume that the Yb^{+3} is located at the same position as the Ca^{+2}, and that the coordinates of the proton nuclei can be calculated, based upon the coordinates of atoms observed by

X-ray crystallographic methods, using standard C-H and N-H bond lengths, and C-C-H and C-N-H bond angles.) There are five unknowns [17] — three to describe the orientation of the principal axis system and the two parameters A_1 and A_2. We will describe the orientation of the principal axis system in terms of the direction cosines L_1, L_2, and L_3 (with $L_1 + L_2 + L_3 = 1$), relative to the X-ray axis system, of a rotation axis and a rotation angle α for the transformation of the coordinates of the protons from the X-ray structure axis system to the new axis system. This set of three unknowns will be represented as (L_1, L_2, α).

III. EXPERIMENTAL PROCEDURES

A. NMR Procedures

^{1}H NMR spectra were obtained on a Bruker HXS-270 spectrometer operating in the Fourier transform mode with quadrature detection. The standard Hahn spin echo pulse sequence, $\pi/2$ - τ - π - τ - acquisition, where tau is equal to 25 ms, was used to accumulate data for the proton NMR spectra shown in Figures 2 and 5. Typical instrumental settings for these spectra were acquisition time 0.8 sec, sweep width +/- 2.5 KHz, spectrum size 8192 data points, and 1 Hz linebroadening. Residual HDO was saturated using the pulsed homonuclear decoupling sequence. The sample temperature was 303°K. The ^{1}H NMR chemical shifts were measured relative to the principal resonance of DSS (2,2-dimethyl-2-silapentane-5-sulfonate) as an internal standard. The standard filters on the HXS-270 spectrometer were replaced with Bessel filters (Ithaco, model 4302).

The ^{19}F spectra were obtained at 254 MHz using the same spectrometer. Typical settings include 0.8 sec acquisition time, sweep width +/- 2.5 KHz, spectrum size 8192 data points, and 5 Hz linebroadening. The sample temperature was 303°K. The ^{19}F chemical shifts were measured relative to 10 mM trifluoroacetic acid in D^{2}0, pH 7.

B. Sample Preparation

Stock ytterbium solutions were prepared from dried Johnson-Matthey ultrapure oxides as discussed earlier [18]. The Yb^{+3} concentrations were determined by titration with EDTA in pH 6 MES (2-(N-morpholino) ethanesulfonic acid) using xylenol orange as an indicator. Microliter ali-

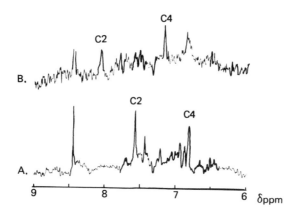

Figure 2. The downfield portion of the 270 MHz ^{1}H NMR spectrum of carp parvalbumin:
A. 0.85 mM calcium saturated carp parvalbumin in 15 mM Pipes, 0.15 M KCl, 0.5 mM DSS, 10 mM DTT, in D_2O, pH 6.35, temperature = 303°K.
B. 0.86 mM parvalbumin in 15 mM Pipes, 0.15 M KCl, 0.5 mM DSS, 10 mM DTT, in D_2O, pH 6.28, temperature = 303°K at a total Yb^{+3} to total protein ratio (Yb/P) of 0.80. The symbols C2 and C4 indicate the resonances of protons bonded to carbons C2 and C4 respectively on histidine 26. These spectra were collected by a $\pi/2 - \tau - \pi - \tau -$ acquisition pulse sequence as described in the Experimental Procedures section.

quots of a Yb^{+3} solution prepared at pH 6.6 were added directly to the protein solution in the NMR tube. The addition did not affect the pH of the resulting protein solution.

Carp parvalbumin (pI=4.25) was isolated by the method of Pechere et al. [19]. The purity and identity of this isotype was confirmed by slab gel electrophoresis, ultraviolet absorption spectra, and amino acid analysis. The fluorinated protein was the gift of Drs. K. Bose and A. Bothner-By. The one sulfhydryl of carp parvalbumin, cysteine 18, was chemically modified by the reagent 2-trifluoroacetoxymercuri-4-fluorophenol.

The NMR samples were prepared by dissolving the lyophilized protein in the standard D^2O buffer consisting of 15 mM Pipes, 0.15 M KCl, 10 mM DTT, 0.5 mM DSS, pH 6.6. pH measurements were made with an Ingold microelectrode (model 6030-04) attached to a Beckman Ex-pandomatic SS-2 or Radiometer 26 pH meter. The pH values quoted are those observed and are not corrected for the deuterium isotope effect. Protein concentrations were determined by amino acid analysis after 24 h of acid hydrolysis at 110°C.

C. Histidine Titration Analysis

Since the protonation of the histidine is in the fast exchange limit, the observed chemical shift is the sum of the protonated [δ_{AH}] and unprotonated [δ_A] chemical shifts, weighted by their respective fractional populations ($f_{AH} + f_A = 1$).

$$\delta_{OBS} = \delta_A (1 - f_{AH}) + f_{AH} (f_{AH})$$

We can rearrange the above equation to the following form:

$$\delta_{OBS} = \delta_A + (\delta_{AH} - \delta_A) \left\{ \frac{[AH]}{[A] + [AH]} \right\}$$

We were unable to titrate His-26 of carp parvalbumin to a low enough pH to observe the fully protonated form since the pKa is quite low (≈ 5) and when the pH approached the isoelectric point (4.25) of the protein it started to come out of solution. We are interested, however, in only the deprotonated shift in the presence and absence of Yb^{+3}. Therefore for the analysis we have assumed ($\delta_{AH} - \delta_A$) to be equal to standard values of 0.93 ppm and 0.42 ppm for the C2 and C4 histidine protons, respectively, [20,21]. The observed values of δ_A for the C2 and C4 protons are quite close to standard values indicating a relatively normal and exposed histidine, supporting the above assumptions.

For the simple deprotonation, AH$\leftrightarrow$H + A, Ka is equal to (H) (A)/(AH). The above equation simplifies to:

$$\delta_{OBS} = \delta_A + (\delta_{AH} - \delta_A) \left\{ \frac{[H]}{Ka + [H]} \right\}$$

The pH titration data were fitted by nonlinear least squares methods to this equation, resulting in values for both Ka and (δ_A).

IV. RESULTS

A. Titrations of Histidine 26

The C2 and C4 protons of His-26 of calcium saturated carp parvalbumin are preferentially observed in the Hahn spin echo spectra shown in Figure 2A because of their relatively narrow linewidths in comparison with the phenylalanine and NH resonances. They were further identified as histidine C2 and C4 protons by their standard chemical shifts [20,21], the fact that they are the only peaks in this region whose chemical shift is pH dependent over the range pH 5-8, and the fact that the C2 proton shifts more (downfield) than the C4 proton as a function of pH (see Figures 3 and 4). These peaks were similarly identified in the spectrum of the protein with Yb^{+3} added to a level where the ratio of total Yb^{+3} to total protein, Yb/P, was 0.80 (Figures 2A, 3, and 4). We have shown elsewhere [10] that up to a ratio of Yb/P of 1/1, the Yb^{+3} has replaced only the Ca^{+2}

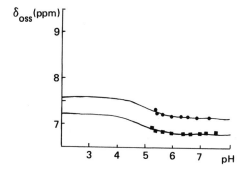

Figure 3. The pH titration curves of the C4 protons of histidine 26 of carp parvalbumin in the presence of saturating levels of calcium (■) and in the presence of Yb^{+3} (●) at a total Yb^{+3} to total protein ratio of 0.80.

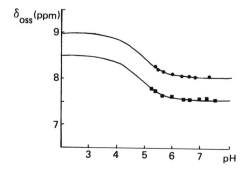

Figure 4. The pH titration curves of the C2 protons of histidine 26 of carp parvalbumin in the presence of saturating levels of calcium (■) and in the presence of Yb^{+3} (●) at a total Yb^{+3} to total protein ratio of 0.80.

bound to the EF hand of parvalbumin. The changes in chemical shift observed, which are presented in Table I, therefore, represent the shifts caused by the Yb^{+3} substituted in the EF calcium binding site. Also presented in Figures 3 and 4 are the least squares fits obtained with the assumptions described in the Experimental Procedures section. The pKa's obtained are presented in Table I.

B.   Observation of the Proton NMR Resonances of the N-acetyl Terminus

The ^{1}H NMR spectrum of the acetyl resonance of carp parvalbumin is shown in Figure 5a. This spectrum was obtained using the Hahn spin echo sequence, and the acetyl protons are again preferentially observed because of their relatively narrow linewidth. The peak at 2.050 ppm relative to DSS has been previously assigned to the N-acetyl resonance, and the peak at 1.90 ppm results from the presence of acetate ions in the sample. For comparison, Parello et al. [22] observe a chemical shift relative to DSS at 2.13 ppm for the N-acetyl resonances and at 1.98 ppm for the acetate resonance. The addition of Yb^{+3} to a total Yb^{+3} to total protein ratio of 0.80, results in both a free and bound resonance for the N-acetyl protons as shown in Figure 5b. This further demonstrates that the metal exchange rates are in the NMR slow exchange limit. A bound chemical shift of 2.083 ppm is observed.

TABLE I

Least Squares Analyses of the NMR pH Titration Data for the C2 and C4 Protons of Histidine 26 of Carp Parvalbumin

Proton	Metal Occupancy		pKa	δ_A (ppm)
	CD	EF		
C2	Ca^{+2}	Ca^{+3}	4.75	7.553
	Ca^{+2}	Yb^{+3}	4.82	8.038
C4	Ca^{+2}	Ca^{+2}	4.80	6.810
	Ca^{+2}	Yb^{+3}	5.00	7.159

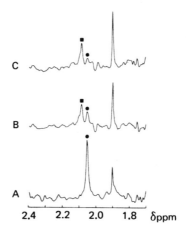

Figure 5. The 270 MHz ^{1}H NMR spectrum of the N-acetyl terminus of carp parvalbumin:

A. 0.85 mM, calcium saturated carp parvalbumin in the standard D$_2$0 buffer, pH 6.72, temperature = 301°K.

B. 0.86 mM carp parvalbumin in the standard D$_2$0 buffer pH 6.72, temperature = 301°K, at a total Yb^{+3} to total protein ratio of 0.80.

C. 0.85 mM carp parvalbumin in the standard D$_2$0 buffer, pH 6.77, temperature = 301°K, at a Yb^{+3} to total protein ratio of 1.05. These spectra were acquired using a $\pi/2 - \tau - \pi - \tau$ - acquisition pulse sequence. The circles (●) indicate the free N-acetyl resonance; the squares (■) indicates the bound resonance.

C. Observation Of The Fluorine NMR Resonance of Fluorinated Carp Parvalbumin

The sulfhydryl of cysteine 18 of carp parvalbumin has been chemically modified with 2-trifluoroacetoxmercuri-4-fluorophenol (see Figure 6 insert). The ^{19}F NMR spectrum of the fluorinated protein is shown in Figure 6. In the presence of calcium, a free chemical shift of -49.541 ppm relative to a standard of 10 mM trifluoroacetic acid in D$_2$0 pH 7 is observed. When Yb^{+3} is added to a total Yb^{+3} to total protein ratio of 0.66, a resonance representing the fluorine label of the protein with Yb^{+3} bound in the EF Ca^{+2} binding site is observed; its chemical shift is -49.381 ppm (Figure 6b). This represents a paramagnetic chemical shift ($\delta_p = \delta_{OBS} - \delta_d$) 0.16 ppm, where δ_{OBS} refers to the observed chemical shift in the presence of the paramagnetic ion, Yb^{+3}, and where δ_d refers to the observed chemical shift in the presence of the diamagnetic ion, Ca^{+2}.

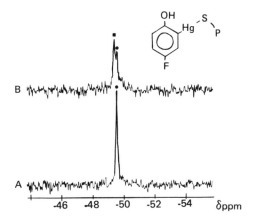

Figure 6. The 254 MHz ^{19}F NMR spectrum of carp parvalbumin chemically modified at cysteine 18 with the reagent 2-trifluoroacetoxymercuri-4-fluorophenol (see insert, the P refers to the protein):
A. 0.84 mM fluorinated parvalbumin in 15 mM Pipes, 0.15 M KCl, 0.5 mM DSS, in D$_2$0, pH 6.67, temperature = 301°K.
B. 0.82 mM fluorinated parvalbumin in 15 mM Pipes, 0.15 M KCl, 0.5 mM DSS, in D$_2$0, pH 6.65, temperature = 301°K at a Yb^{+3} to total protein ratio of 0.66. The chemical shift is measured with respect to 10 mM trifluoroacetic acid in D20, pH 7. The circles (●) indicate the free fluorine resonance. The squares (■) indicates the bound fluorine resonance.

V. DISCUSSION

We have outlined elsewhere the strategy for the complete analysis of the lanthanide induced ^{1}H NMR chemical shifts of the ytterbium-parvalbumin complex in order to determine the three dimensional structure of the EF binding site of carp parvalbumin in solution [10]. In this paper, we discuss the assignment of the resonances of the C2 and C4 protons of histidine, of the N-acetylated terminus, and of a sulfhydryl specific fluorinated reporter group, bound to the protein. We also discuss the determination of their paramagnetic chemical shifts and their role in the analysis of the NMR data.

Lanthanide induced ^{1}H NMR shifts have been used previously to probe the structure of lysozyme and the bovine pancreatic trypsin inhibitor [14,17,23-25]. Neither of these proteins have high affinity specific metal binding sites. In both these examples the ^{1}H NMR spectra are in the fast exchange limit. This has the advantage that assigned resonances may be followed as a function of metal concentration. It has, however, the disadvantage that shifts and linewidths or relaxation rates have to be extrapolated to infinite metal concentrations to determine the shifts and relaxation rates characterizing the protein-metal ion complex and nonspecific binding can influence the results at the high concentrations of metal ion required. In our case, the protein has high affinity specific metal binding sites which result in spectra in the NMR slow exchange limit. The advantage here is that the chemical shifts and relaxation rates of the parvalbumin-paramagnetic ion complex may be accurately and directly determined.

The substitution of calcium by ytterbium at a Yb/P ratio of 0.80 results in a series of shifted resonances in the NMR slow exchange limit. By analogy to X-ray crystallographic data [26] and optical studies [27,28], we conclude that the substitution occurs initially in the EF site [10]. (At higher ratios of Yb/P, a new series of peaks arise [10,16]. The analysis of the stoichiometry of binding of ytterbium to the two sites of parvalbumin will be presented in detail elsewhere [32]).

The C2 and C4 resonances of histidine 26 were followed as a function of pH (Figures 3 and 4). At low pH's, the shifts could not accurately be determined, due to the isoelectric precipitation of this parvalbumin (pI = 4.25). The pKa's for the histidine are listed in Table I. These unusually low pKa's ($\approx$4.8) may result from the presence of a nearby positive charge, lysine 27. In addition to the pKa of histidine, least squares analyses have resulted in the determination of (δ_A) for the C2 and C4 protons, 7.553 ppm and 6.816 ppm respectively. In the presence of Yb^{+3} at a total Yb^{+3} to total protein ratio of 0.80, these resonances have shifted significantly (Figures 3 and 4). The calculated pKa's do not differ, but the observed chemical shifts do. The chemical shifts (δ_A) for the C2 and C4 protons in the presence of Yb^{+3} are 8.038 and 7.159 ppm respectively. This represents downfield paramagnetic shifts of 0.485 ppm for the C2 proton and 0.343 ppm for the C4 protons. The paramagnetic shift of the N-acetyl terminus of 0.033 ppm has also been determined (Figure 5). Since both the free and the bound resonances are observed, we can calculate the minimum lifetime of the ytterbium on the protein as 18 ms.

We now need to find the orientation of the principal axis system of the magnetic susceptibility tensor and the elements A_1 and A_2 in order that we may calculate shifts from the structure using Equation 1. This requires the determination of five unknowns; (L_1, L_2, α) and A_1, A_2. We only have three assigned resonances with measured shifts whose position we can calculate from the X-ray structure, which is not sufficient. We have a measured shift for the fluorine label but do not know its position in the protein with certainty, so we will reserve it for a check on our final calculations. We need other resonances to aid our determination of principal axis system.

One useful set is the six shifted methyl resonances which were identified by their area [10], since there are a total of only seven methyls within 10 Å of the EF metal binding site. Two of these methyls are shifted more downfield than 10 ppm, and appear at 17.79 ppm ($\delta_p = 17.69$ ppm) and 15.17 ppm ($\delta_p = 14.17$ ppm) in Figure 1. The other four observed methyls are shifted upfield, the most upfield shifted appearing at -1.59 ppm ($\delta_p = 1.90$ ppm). Two of these upfield shifted methyls are seen overlapping at $\delta = -1.6$ ppm in Figure 1b. The chemical shifts for these methyl groups are listed in Table III.

We also need to know the coordinates of the protons surrounding the metal in order to calculate spectra based upon the known X-ray structure. The last Diamond refined X-ray structure of parvalbumin [29] was chosen as the most appropriate starting point. Proton coordinates were generated from this structure assuming standard bond lengths and geometries. In the case of methyl groups, the "methyl proton centroid" model [30] was used to determine the average methyl proton positions.

The shifts of these three assigned resonances were then used in conjunction with the methyl group shifts to determine the NMR unknowns. The search for the best fit solution to the NMR unknowns was made in the following manner. For a given choice of (L_1, L_2, α), the geometric factors G_1 and G_2 were calculated for the His C2, His C4 and N-acetyl CH_3 protons. The parameters A_1 and A_2 for this particular choice of axis system were then taken as those giving the best least squares fit of the calculated shifts to the observed shifts for these nuclei. If the resultant calculated shifts for the assigned resonances were in good agreement with the observed shifts, the shifts of the CH_3 groups near the EF site were then calculated from their geometry in this axis system and the best fit A_1 and A_2. The choice of axis system was then rejected if it did not meet the criteria of having only 2 methyl groups shifted more downfield than 10 ppm, and having no methyl resonance shifted more upfield than -5 ppm. If the solution passed the above criteria, the goodness of the solution was tested by calculating a chi value comparing the two calculated most downfield methyl shifts with the observed values of $\delta_p = 17.69$ and 14.17 ppm, and the calculated most upfield methyl shift with the observed $\delta_p = 1.9$ ppm. One best fit solution was identified on the basis of the best fit of the calculated shifts to the His C2, His C4 and N-acetyl shifts and the three shifted methyls discussed above. In fact, 24 solutions were found corresponding to the various possible permutations of the labelling of the principal axis system [24], and the final solution selected by adopting the convention that $\|A_1\|$ be maximal, and that $0 < \|A_2/A_1\| < 1$. In this regard the fact that these assigned nuclei are relatively far removed from the metal turned out to be an advantage because their calculated geometric factors, G_1 and G_2 from Equation (1), were not sensitive to inaccuracies in the X-ray structure. The histidines and the N-acetyl nuclei are also situated at diverse angular orientations which is advantageous for the fitting procedure. The values for the best fit solution are $L_1 = -0.60$, $L_2 = -0.77$, $L_3 = -0.217$, and $\alpha = 4.11$ radians, with the values of A^1 and A^2 equal to -5450 ppm A^{+3} and -3360 ppm A^{+3}, respectively.

The calculated shifts of the His 26 C2, His 26 C4 and N-acetyl protons from the best fit solution obtained in the manner described above are listed in Table II. There is excellent agreement between the calculated and observed results here, indicated by a standard deviation of ± 0.008 ppm. The paramagnetic shifts for the observed methyl groups and the distances obtained from their linewidths are listed in Table III. Also listed are the best fit calculated shifts, and the distances based upon the X-ray structure, for the seven methyl groups within 10 Å of the EF binding site. One can see that there is fair agreement for the two most downfield shifted methyl groups (17.69 vs 18.075) and (14.17 vs 11.297). In addition the predicted distances to the metal (6.1 and 9.0 Å) correspond well with the observed distances (6.2 ± 0.2 and 7.9 + 1.8/-0.7 Å) which were calculated from the linewidths of these resonances [11]. However there is less agreement between the observed and calculated chemical shifts for the remaining five methyls.

A list of the most downfield and most upfield observed and calculated shifts is presented in Table IV. The six most downfield observed shifts are in the range of 18.90 to 27.62 ppm. Three resonances with shifts greater than 27.62 ppm are calculated. The six most upfield shifted resonances have observed chemical shifts of -12.68 to -19.06 ppm. Sixteen resonances with chemical shifts more upfield than -19.06 ppm are predicted. Also indicated in Table IV is the predicted linewidth of the shifted resonances relative to the linewidth of the peak at 29.80 ppm. This calculation is based upon a r^6 dependence of the linewidth and a calculated distance from the observed linewidth of 5.9 Å for the peak at 19.80 ppm.

The result of our NMR fitting procedure is that we are able to choose a set of parameters which give calculated NMR shifts which fit the observed shifts of the assigned His 26 C2, His 26 C4, and N-acetyl methyl resonances quite well. These resonances are far removed (13-20 Å) from the metal ion so that there is no possibility of a contact contribution to the shifts, and small errors in the X-ray structure such as the less well defined

TABLE II

Chemical Shift Data of the Assigned Histidine and N-Acetyl Resonances of Parvalbumin

Nucleus	Observed[a] δ_p	Calculated δ_p	$r(\overset{\circ}{A})^b$
His 26 C2	0.485	0.488	13.6
His 26 C4	0.343	0.337	15.1
N-Acetyl	0.033	0.042	20.1

a   Chemical shifts are measured in ppm.
b   Calculated from X-ray structure [29].
Source: From Ref. 10.

TABLE III

A Comparison of the Observed and Calculated Chemical Shifts and Distances for the Seven Methyl Groups Within 10 Å of the EF Site

Observed δ_p[a]	$r(\overset{\circ}{A})^b$	Calculated δ_p[a]	Nucleus	$r(\overset{\circ}{A})^e$
17.690	6.2 + 0.2/-0.2	18.075	Leu 86 δ 1	6.1
14.170	7.9 + 1.8/-0.7	11.297	Val 99 γ 2	9.0
c	d	9.807	Ile 97 γ 2	6.0
-0.365	d	6.270	Ile 97 δ 1	7.2
-1.440	d	6.120	Leu 86 δ 2	8.4
-1.621	d	-1.037	Ile 58 δ 1	10.2
-1.900	d	-3.793	Ile 58 γ 2	9.6

a   Ranked in order of decreasing shift in ppm (from Reference 10).
b   Calculated from linewidths [11].
c   Not shifted outside the diamagnetic spectrum.
d   The field dependence of the linewidths has not been determined.
e   Calculated from X-ray structure [29].
Source: From Ref. 10.

TABLE IV

A Comparison of the Most Upfield and Most Downfield Observed Calculated Chemical Shifts

Observed δp	Calculated δ_p	Nucleus	Relative broadening[a]
	47.473	Asp 90 β	3.50
	35.455	Glu 101 β	2.71
	32.949	Asp 94 β	3.66
27.62	27.191	Gly 95 α	0.64
25.77	26.634	Asp 90 β	1.36
22.26	26.011	Gly 93 α	1.69
22.09	25.914	Asp 94 α	0.78
20.10	24.024	Ile 97 γ	3.64
18.90	17.618	Glu 101 γ	4.41
-12.86	-13.332	Phe 57 α	0.25
-14.16	-13.536	Lys 96 ϵ	0.10
-14.53	-13.628	Glu 59 γ	0.08
-14.60	-17.281	Lys 96 ϵ	0.12
-16.20	-17.921	Phe 57 β	0.14
-19.06	-20.128	Asp 92 β	3.81
	-28.628	Lys 96 δ	0.59
	-28.814	Ser 91 α	0.44
	-29.154	Ser 91 β	0.29
	-30.477	Lys 96 γ	0.59
	-31.068	Glu 101 γ	3.91
	-33.090	Phe 57 β	0.44
	-35.307	Asp 92 α	1.01
	-39.388	Lys 96 δ	0.68
	-40.338	Lys 96 γ	0.59
	-41.793	Lys 96 α	2.12
	-50.889	Asp 92 β	4.83
	-53.348	Phe 57 ϵ	14.11
	-57.797	Ser 91 β	1.25
	-95.357	Phe 57 δ	3.98
	-119.548	Lys 96 β	8.60
	-148.459	Lys 96 β	7.46

a   This column indicates the predicted linebroadening relative to the linewidth of the resonances with δ_{OBS} of 29.80 ppm and r=5.85 Å (which was calculated from its linewidth); this predicted line broadening is based on a r^6 dependence (See Theory Section).

Source: From Ref. 10.

electron density in the region of the amino terminus are not going to greatly influence the calculated shifts. Also the diamagnetic positions of these resonances were independently determined. Therefore we feel that our choice of best fit is not ambiguous, nor are any of the assumptions made likely to be incorrect for these resonances.

We have measured the chemical shift for the fluorine label which also fits the above criteria, but do not know its exact location. Using the best fit values of L_1, L_2, α, A_1 and A_2 as listed above, we are able to predict a paramagnetic chemical shift for this label, if we assume its position to be equivalent to the position of the sulfur atom of cysteine 18. The predicted value for the paramagnetic chemical shift is 0.182 ppm which is comparable to the observed value of 0.16 ppm. This serves to confirm our determination of L_1, L_2, α, A_1, and A_2.

As we move in toward the metal ion, the agreement between the calculated and observed spectra gets worse. The situation is fair for the methyl groups which are 6-11 Å from the metal ion especially considering potential inaccuracies in the determination of the diamagnetic shifts and the use of the "centroid" model for the average methyl proton position. The calculated and observed distances agree quite well as an additional indication of the correctness of the best fit solution.

The agreement between calculated and observed shifts is very poor, however, for the nuclei close to the metal. Indeed we were not able to find any fit based upon reasonable criteria which did not give calculated shifts way outside the range of the observed shifts. While it is possible that some nearby nuclei are shifted outside of the observed range and also broadened beyond detection (see relative linewidth prediction in Table IV), and it might be possible that some very nearby nuclei have compensating contact shifts, neither explanation could account for a large number of the nuclei which are calculated to have very large shifts. Another potential problem is internal motions in the protein. One would expect, however, the observed NMR shifts to be too large rather than too small reflecting an unequal weighting of closer conformations in averages of the sort of $<1/r^{+3}>$. We feel that the biggest source of error is inaccuracies in the X-ray based proton coordinates at a level below the resolution of the X-ray method (1.9 Å in this case). That is, errors of the order of 0.5 Å in the position of nuclei as close as 3-4 Å, while not detectable in the X-ray method, greatly influence the NMR results. We hope to generate a refined structure with the aid of the NMR data at a level of resolution presently unobtainable by X-ray methods.

The orientation of ligands in the EF calcium binding site of carp parvalbumin in the principal axis system of the magnetic susceptibility tensor of the metal ion is shown as a stereodiagram in Figure 7a. An examination of this arrangement of oxygen atoms (Figure 7b) reveals that the coordination resembles a distorted trigonal antiprism with the Z axis intercepting the opposite trigonal faces. Few examples of the geometry of 6 coordinate lanthanide complexes are available for comparison, however; and the question remains as to the participation of some of the other carbonyl oxygens in metal coordination [26]. The exact structure of the ligands around the Yb^{+3} in the principal axis system of the magnetic susceptibility tensor must, therefore, await for refinement of the structure.

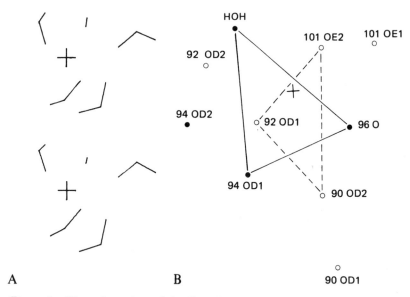

A   B   90 OD1

Figure 7.   The orientation of the ligands in the EF metal binding site of carp parvalbumin in the principal axis system of the magnetic susceptibility tensor of the ytterbium ion:

A. A stereodiagram of the oxygen ligands in the EF metal binding site. The origin is at the metal ion position. The positive Z axis is pointed out of the page, the positive Y axis is vertical and the positive X axis points to the right.

B. A projection of the oxygen atoms in the EF metal binding site in the XY plane. The origin is at the metal ion position. The positive Z axis is pointed out of the page, the positive Y axis is vertical, and the positive X axis points to the right. Reference 6 contains the atom nomenclature designations. Those atoms represented by open circles (O) are in the positive Z direction, above the plan of the paper; those atoms represented by filled circles (●) are in the negative Z direction, below the plane of the paper. The values of Z are listed below (in Å): (HOH, -1.0; 90-OD2, 1.2; 90-0D1, 0.2; 92-0D2, 0.8; 92-OD1, 1.7; 94-0D2, -1.9; 94-0D1, -1.2; 96-0, -1.4; 101-0E2, 2-0; 101-0E1, 0.3).

Figure 7, however, seems stereochemically reasonable and, therefore, is a suggestive indicator that we have properly located .the principal axis system.

Acknowledgments

We acknowledge many helpful discussions with Dr. Timothy D. Marinetti and with Dr. Edward R. Birnbaum, whose initial observation of the lanthanide shifted resonances of the troponin C CB-9-Pr^{+3} complex [31] lead to much of this present work. We thank Drs. K. Bose and A. Bothner-By for their very generous gift of the fluorine labelled parvalbumin. We acknowledge the assistance of Drs. Louis Delbaere and Brian F. P. Edwards in calculating the X-ray based proton coordinates. We also thank Colin Broughton for preparing the stereo diagram in Figure 7. This work was supported by the Medical Research Council of Canada Group on Protein Structure and Function.

References

1. R. H. Kretsinger, *Ann. Rev. of Biochem., 45*:239 (1976).
2. H. Rasmussen, D. B. P. Goodman, and A. Tenehouse, *C.R.C. Crit. Rev. Biochem., 1*:95 (1972).
3. J. D. Potter, J. D. Johnson, J. R. Dedman, W. E. Schreiber, F. Mandel, R. L. Jackson, and A. R. Means in *Calcium Binding Proteins and Calcium Function*, (R. J. Wasserman, R. A. Corradino, E. Carafoli, R. H. Kretsinger, D. H. MacLennan, and F. L. Siegel, eds.), Elsevier, New York, 1977, p. 239.
4. A. Weeds, P. Wagner, R. Jakes, and J. Kendrick-Jones in *Calcium Binding Proteins and Calcium Function* (R. J. Wasserman, R. A. Corradino, E. Carafoli, R. H. Kretsinger, D. H. MacLennan, and F. L. Siegel, eds.) Elsevier, New York, 1977, p. 222.
5. F. C. Stevens, M. Walsh, H. C. Ho, T. S. Teo, and J. H. Wang, *J. Biol. Chem., 251*:4495 (1976).
6. R. H. Kretsinger and C. E. Nockolds, *J. Biol. Chem., 248*:3313 (1973).
7. A. G. Weeds and A. D. MacLachlan, *Nature, 252*:646 (1974).
8. J. H. Collins, *Biochem., Biophys. Res. Commun., 58*:301 (1974).
9. J. H. Collins, *Nature, 259*:699 (1976).
10. L. Lee and B. D. Sykes, *Biophys. J., 32*:193 (1980).
11. L. Lee and B. D. Sykes, *Biochem., 19*:3208 (1980).
12. B. Bleaney, *J. Magn. Reson., 8*:91 (1972).
13. J. M. Briggs, G. P. Moss, E. W. Randall, and K. D. Sales, *J. Chem. Soc. Chem. Commun.*, p. 1180 (1972).
14. T. D. Marinetti, G. H. Snyder, and B. D. Sykes, *J. Amer. Chem. Soc., 97*:6562 (1975).
15. J. Reuben, *J. Magn. Reson., 11*:103 (1973).

16. L. Lee and B. D. Sykes, *Adv. Inorg. Biochem., 2*:183 (1980).
17. T. D. Marinetti, G. H. Snyder, and B. D. Sykes, *Biochem., 16*:647 (1977).
18. E. R. Birnbaum and B. D. Sykes, *Biochem., 17*:4965 (1978).
19. J. F. Pechere, J. Demaille, and J. P. Capony, *Biochim. Biophys. Acta, 236*:391 (1971).
20. J. L. Markley, *Accts. Chem. Res., 8*:70 (1975).
21. B. F. P. Edwards and B. D. Sykes, *Biochem., 17*:684 (1978).
22. J. Parello, A. Cave, P. Puigdomenech, C. Maury, J. P. Capony, and J. F. Pechere, *Biochim., 56*:61 (1974).
23. I. D. Campbell, C. M. Dobson, and R. J. P. Williams, *Proc. R. Soc. Lond. A., 345*:41 (1975).
24. D. G. Agresti, R. E. Lenkinski, and J. D. Glickson, *Biochem. Biophys. Res. Comm., 76*:711 (1977).
25. T. D. Marinetti, G. H. Snyder, and B. D. Sykes, *Biochem., 15*:4600 (1976).
26. J. Sowadski, G. Cornick, and R. H. Kretsinger, *J. Mol. Biol., 124*:123 (1978).
27. W. DeW. Horrocks, Jr. and D. R. Sudnick, *J. Amer. Chem. Soc., 101*:334 (1979).
28. H. Donato, Jr. and R. B. Martin, *Biochem., 33*:445 (1979).
29. P. C. Moews and R. H. Kretsinger, *J. Mol. Biol., 91*:201 (1975).
30. R. Rowan III, J. A. McGammon, and B. D. Sykes, *J. Amer. Chem. Soc., 96*:4773 (1974).
31. L. Lee, B. D. Sykes and E. R. Birnbaum, *FEBS Lett., 98*:169 (1979).
32. L. Lee and B. D. Sykes, *Biochem., 20*:0000 (1981).

CHAPTER 8

STRUCTURAL STUDIES ON HIGH AFFINITY CALCIUM BINDING PROTEINS: SKELETAL TROPONIN-C AND BRAIN CALMODULIN

Kenneth B. Seamon
Laboratory of Bioorganic Chemistry
National Institute of Arthritis, Metabolism, and Digestive Diseases
National Institutes of Health
Bethesda, Maryland

I. INTRODUCTION

A. Physiologic Role of Calcium and Calcium "Receptor" Proteins

Calcium has been shown to play an integral role in regulating numerous cellular events including stimulus-secretion coupling [1], cellular motility [2], muscle contraction [3], steroidogenesis [4], as well as a number of other diverse physiological responses (for a review see reference 5). The importance of calcium in regulating nerve cell function has been long recognized [6]. It has been postulated that calcium may act alone or in concert with cyclic nucleotides in the role of a second messenger [7]. Furthermore, calcium has been shown to be involved in the regulation of presynaptic [8] and postsynaptic events in neuronal cells [9].

Increases in intracellular calcium are the result of cellular excitation via either chemically or electrically induced membrane depolarization or possibly by an indirect effect of cyclic nucleotides. The increased intracellular calcium could be due to release from intracellular storage sites such as mitochondria or sarcoplasmic reticular membranes in cardiac cells. Alternatively, the increased calcium could be the result of an accelerated influx of calcium from the extracellular medium where the calcium concentration is high, 2-3mM.

In order for calcium to exert its regulatory effects the transient increase in free calcium must be recognized by some component of the target enzyme system. The recognition process involves calcium binding proteins [10] which are the initial molecular target for calcium; e.g., troponin-C, calmodulin. These proteins have calcium binding sites with dissociation constants between $10^{-8}M$-$10^{-6}M$ such that the sites are unoccupied in the unstimulated cell but bind calcium when the intracellular calcium increases in the stimulated cell. After binding calcium the calcium binding protein must be able to transmit the message of its bound calcium ion to an associated enzyme system. This is accomplished by a Ca^{2+}-induced conformational change in the binding protein. This conformational change can be transmitted to other cellular components by: 1) a further conformational change induced in proteins that do not bind calcium but are bound to the calcium receptor protein; e.g., troponin-I and troponin-T in the muscle regulatory system [11,12]; 2) the unmasking of regions of the receptor protein which are able to interact with other protein components leading to complex formation, e.g., calmodulin interactions with phosphodiesterase [13] and adenylate cyclase [14]; and 3) the unmasking of hydrophobic regions of the receptor protein allowing it to interact with membranes; e.g., S-100 [15] and possibly calmodulin [16]. The primary event in all of the above phenomenon is the initial binding of calcium and a concomittant or subsequent conformational change that occurs in the calcium receptor protein.

B. Structural Considerations for Homologous Calcium Binding Proteins

Studies by Kretsinger and associates and others on the crystal structure of carp-parvalbumin, a low molecular weight calcium binding protein, and its sequence homology with other high affinity calcium binding proteins have provided a framework for discussing the tertiary structure of these so called "EF-hand" calcium binding proteins [17-20]. The term "EF-hand" refers to the structural unit which defines a calcium binding domain. This domain consists of a binding loop of twelve amino acid residues, containing six residues which participate in coordinating calcium, and two turns of α-helix flanking both sides of the binding loop. It has been proposed that high affinity calcium regulatory proteins have evolved with similar binding sites consisting of an EF-hand [21]. The EF-hand, and therefore putative binding sites, can be identified in a number of calcium binding proteins by their homologous sequences with the model calcium binding domain derived from the structure of carp-parvalbumin [22]. This concept has proved to be extremely valuable in discussing the tertiary structure of these proteins since until recently it has proved difficult to produce crystals of these proteins (except for carp-parvalbumin) suitable for structure determination by x-ray crystallography.

1. Carp-parvalbumin

Carp-parvalbumin has a molecular weight of 11,500 and binds two moles of calcium with high affinity [23]. Calcium is bound at two similar binding sites, the CD and EF sites, which are structurally related by an approximate two-fold symmetry axis. The two binding sites along with the associated helical regions are illustrated in Figure 1. The binding site geometry is best described as an approximately octahedral coordination of calcium with a water molecule occupying one of the vertices in the EF loop. A more detailed discussion of the tertiary structure of carp-parvalbumin is presented elsewhere in this volume and only a few salient points will be mentioned here. The conformation of the calcium saturated protein is characteristic of a soluble globular protein with a well defined hydrophobic core consisting of nonpolar amino acid residues [17]. The solution conformation of the calcium saturated protein and apo-protein have been studied using NMR [24-27]. The results are most consistent with the calcium saturated conformation being very structured with few, if any, regions of random coil structure. The interior of the protein contains sidechains from phenylalanine residues, some of which occur at positions in the helical regions adjacent to the binding loops. It is easy to envision how structural alterations at the binding site, due to calcium binding and neutralization of negative-charges, could affect the adjacent helical regions. This structural modification could then lead to a change in the interaction of the phenylalanine residues in the interior of the protein. Thus, it is feasible that a local conformational change in the binding site could be amplified or transmitted to a more distant part of the protein structure.

2. Skeletal Troponin-C

Troponin-C has a molecular weight of *ca.* 18,000 and binds four moles of calcium. The protein is very acidic, pI *ca.* 4.1, with an amino acid composi-

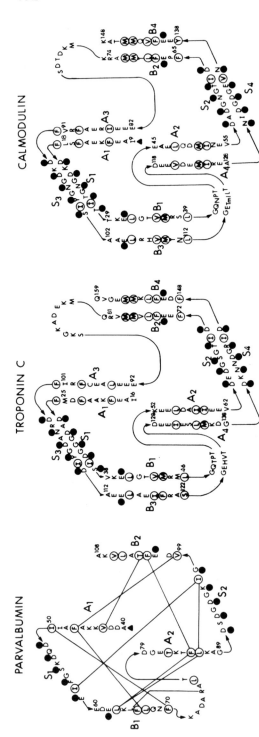

Figure 1. Homologous Binding Domains in Carp-Parvalbumin, Rabbit Skeletal Troponin-C, and Bovine Brain Calmodulin. The sequences of parvalbumin, skeletal troponin-C, and brain calmodulin are aligned and represented as discussed by Weeds and McLachlan [20] for parvalbumin and troponin-C. The binding domains are labeled S₁ through S₄, with associated helical segments A₁-A₄ and B₁-B₄. Residues predicted to participate on calcium coordination are indicated by the filled circles. Those residues that are predicted to take part in hydrophobic interactions in the interior of the protein are circled. Specific hydrophobic interactions in parvalbumin are indicated by lines connecting the amino acid residues in close contact. (Adapted with permission from A. Weeds and A. McLachlan, *Nature*, 252:646 (1974); copyright Macmillan Journals Ltd).

tion characterized by the absence of tryptophan, and the presence of two tyrosines, one histidine, and one cysteine. The complete amino acid sequence has been determined and it has been shown that four "EF-hands", representing the four calcium binding sites, S_1-S_4, can be identified in the sequence [28]. These are depicted in Figure 1. It can be seen that calcium binding ligands as well as hydrophobic amino acid residues appear in homologous positions to those in carp-parvalbumin. The calcium and magnesium binding parameters of troponin-C, determined by Potter and Gergely [29], showed that calcium is bound at two classes of sites, two high affinity sites which can competitively bind magnesium and two lower affinity calcium specific sites.

It is now generally accepted that the S_1 and S_2 sites correspond to the low affinity sites while the S_3 and S_4 sites are the high affinity sites [30,31]. It has also been suggested that the link region between the two pairs of sites, residues 88-119, may represent a site of interaction between troponin-C and troponin-I [32]. Much of this work has relied on the availability of proteolytic fragments of the protein that retain biological activity, e.g., metal binding, binding to troponin-I. These fragments have also been useful in studies relating to the tertiary structure of the whole protein.

Hydrodynamic studies indicate that, like carp-parvalbumin, troponin-C is a globular protein in solution and contains considerable secondary structure, both in the metal free and calcium saturated states [33]. It was demonstrated by a variety of techniques that calcium binding to troponin-C results in a large change in its solution conformation. This conformational change is characterized by the following: 1) an increase in helical content [33,34]; 2) an increase in tyrosine fluorescence [34]; 3) a decreased reactivity of cysteine-98 to chemical modifying agents [35]; and 4) a positive tyrosyl UV difference spectrum [36]. The calcium induced conformational change results not only in alterations in the secondary structure but also in the tertiary structure.

3. Calmodulin

Calmodulin has a molecular weight of *ca.* 16,500 and like troponin-C binds four moles of calcium. Its amino acid composition is very similar to that of troponin-C. Calmodulin contains no cysteine but does contain one mole of the unusual amino acid ϵ-trimethyllysine. The amino acid sequence of calmodulin isolated from a number of mammalian species has been determined and except for a few assignments the sequences are identical [37-39]. Four metal binding domains can be identified in the sequence of calmodulin (see Figure 1) and like those in troponin-C the placement of metal binding ligands in the binding loop and nonpolar amino acid residues in the helical regions are identical to those in carpparvalbumin [40]. These regions most likely correspond to the four calcium binding sites of calmodulin. It has not been unequivocally determined how many classes of binding sites calmodulin has and therefore an exact identification of "high" or "low" affinity sites is not yet possible.

The sequences of troponin-C and calmodulin are very similar with ca. 80% of the 147 residues being either identical or functionally conserved [40]. A consequence of this similarity in sequence is that the two proteins display very similar physical properties [41,42]. Apo-calmodulin contains considerable secondary structure but there appear to be regions of the polypeptide chain that are unfolded in the absence of calcium and are susceptible to proteolytic enzymes [43]. This has also been observed for troponin-C [44]. The physical and chemical indicators of a calcium induced conformational change in calmodulin are similar to those previously described for troponin-C [45]. One notable exception is that calcium induces a negative tyrosyl UV difference spectrum for calmodulin which is attributed to an unusual chemical environment of tyrosine-138.

4. Other EF-Hand Calcium Binding Proteins

A computer search of known protein amino acid sequences revealed a number of proteins that contain regions of partial or complete homology with the model EF-hand calcium binding loop [22]. Some of these proteins are known to contain calcium binding sites while others display little or no calcium binding. It has been recognized, however, that a number of evolutionarily related proteins do exist that contain partial or complete EF-hands.

Cardiac troponin-C is involved in the regulation of cardiac muscle contraction. Although the protein is similar to skeletal troponin-C, it binds only three moles of calcium [46-48]. The amino acid sequence of bovine cardiac troponin-C has been determined and displays ca. 65% identical or functionally conserved homology with skeletal troponin-C [49]. Four regions of the sequence can be identified as calcium binding domains. However, it is observed that the first domain is probably structurally defective with respect to calcium binding. Two of the residues in the first domain that participate directly in the coordination of calcium are aspartic acid residues in the skeletal protein. These are replaced by alanine and leucine residues in the cardiac protein. Based on these substitutions it is predicted that the first binding loop of the cardiac protein is less likely to bind calcium. This observation is consistent with binding data indicating that cardiac troponin-C contains only one calcium specific binding site [46], instead of two as is the case for the skeletal protein, since site 1 in the skeletal protein is a calcium specific site. It has also been demonstrated that cardiac troponin-C undergoes a calcium induced conformational change which is similar to that seen for skeletal troponin-C [50,51].

Calcium binding proteins, whose levels seem to respond to vitamin D or one of its metabolites, have been isolated from intestine. Two forms of these proteins have been described; a 9,700 MW form isolated from mammalian intestine and a second form of 28,000 MW isolated from avian intestinal systems [52]. The sequence of the 9,700 MW protein has been determined and two EF-calcium binding domains can be identified [53]. This is consistent with the report that the protein can bind two moles of calcium, even though one of the calcium binding domains contains a three residue deletion [53]. The protein has considerable secondary structure in the absence of calcium and undergoes a calcium induced change in conformation which is characterized by a decreased sensitivity of the calcium saturated protein to proteolysis [53].

Myosin molecules consist of two large or heavy chains of 200,000 MW and two pairs of light chains with molecular weights of *ca.* 20,000 MW. The light chains are classified as the DTNB light chains and the EDTA light chains [54]. The amino acid sequences of the EDTA light chains from rabbit skeletal muscle have been determined [55] allowing the identification of four calcium binding domains in their respective sequences [20]. Only one of the light chains, the DTNB light chain, binds calcium in its isolated state [56]. It is thought that the EDTA light chains may bind calcium only in their native state associated with myosin. The sequence homology and associated deletions and insertions are discussed in detail elsewhere with respect to the inability of these proteins to bind calcium [57]. Nevertheless they still are considered part of the EF-hand family of calcium binding proteins. Physical studies on the light chains indicate that the isolated chains contain regions of globular structure; however, it appears that they contain larger regions of random coil than the previously described calcium binding proteins [58,59]. The calcium-induced conformational change for the DTNB light chain is qualitatively similar to that seen for troponin-C, but it appears to represent a smaller overall change in protein conformation [59].

The S-100 protein is a nervous system specific protein whose function, although unknown, is postulated to be linked to its ability to bind calcium and monovalent cations [60]. It differs from the other calcium binding proteins previously described in that it exists in solution as a dimer rather than a single polypeptide chain [61,62]. The dimer is composed of a combination of four different subunits each having a molecular weight of *ca.* 10,500, but being structurally and immunologically different [62]. It is not clear whether the native protein exists only as a homogenous dimer of two identical subunits, or a heterogenous dimer consisting of two different subunits. The amino acid sequence of one of the major subunits has been determined and one region of the sequence can be identified as a calcium binding domain [61]. Since the native protein exists as a dimer it would be predicted that S-100 can bind two moles of calcium. This prediction has been confirmed in calcium binding studies performed at low ionic strength [63]. High concentrations of monovalent cations inhibit calcium binding to the S-100 protein. S-100 undergoes a characteristic calcium induced conformational change which affects the environment of a number of its amino acid residues [64]. The conformational change results in the exposure of a hydrophobic region capable of binding the dye, anilinonapthol-sulfonic acid [65], and facilitating the binding of S-100 to synaptic membranes [66]. Although it exhibits many characteristics of the EF-hand calcium binding proteins, the S-100 protein also represents a special class of these proteins due to its native dimeric structure.

C. Scope

Although it is clear that a wide variety of physiologically important calcium binding proteins exist, the scope of this chapter will be limited to the discussion of the two closely related calcium dependent regulatory proteins, skeletal troponin-C and calmodulin. The aim of this chapter is to demonstrate how ^{1}H-NMR techniques have allowed a better understanding of the mechanisms through which the calcium regulatory proteins exert their physiological control. The studies referred to were chosen to address the following questions.

1. What are the solution conformations of the calcium regulatory proteins and how are they modified by metal binding?
2. Are the solution structures of the calcium regulatory proteins, as revealed by NMR, consistent with the observed sequence homology with carp-parvalbumin, and does the sequence homology result in structural homology as well as similarities in the calcium induced conformational change?

II. TROPONIN-C

A. Role of Troponin-C in the Regulation of Striated Muscle

Troponin-C is the calcium receptor protein associated with the troponin regulatory complex of striated muscle. Troponin is situated on the actin thin filament. In the absence of calcium, troponin, along with tropomyosin, inhibits the hydrolysis of ATP by the actin-myosin complex. A transient increase in the free calcium concentration and subsequent formation of a troponin-C calcium complex in the troponin regulatory complex ultimately leads to the release of the inhibition of the actin-myosin ATPase and allows the contractile event to occur [3]. The initial event is the formation of a calcium troponin-C complex which results in a change in the conformation of the protein. Although the exact molecular mechanism has not been established it is presumed that a change in the conformation of troponin-C leads to a change in the orientation of tropomyosin with respect to the actin filament [67]. It is generally agreed however that the binding of calcium to troponin-C is the initial event in the skeletal contractile process.

B. Conformation of Apo-Troponin-C

The ^{1}H-NMR spectrum of the aromatic and aliphatic region of the apo-protein is shown in Figure 2. The ring proton resonances of tyrosines 10 and 109, exhibit the same chemical shifts. In addition, both phenolic moieties have the same pKa of *ca.* 10.4 [68]. The chemical shifts and titration behavior are similar to that of a tyrosine in an aqueous environment and thus suggest that both tyrosines of troponin-C are exposed to solvent. This conclusion is also supported by chemical modification studies on apo-troponin-C [69]. Similarly, it is observed that the bulk of the phenylalanine ring proton resonance intensity is at a chemical shift position (7.34 ppm) characteristic of solvent exposed phenylalanine rings. These results suggest that a large amount of the polypeptide chain is in a random coil configuration with little or no tertiary structure. However, the protein is not in a denatured state as evidenced by the two upfield shifted phenylalanine resonances at 6.44 ppm and 6.67 ppm and the two upfield shifted aliphatic peaks at 0.166 ppm and -.15 ppm. These two sets of resonances indicate that there is a region of structure in the apo-protein which is characterized by close interactions between nonpolar amino

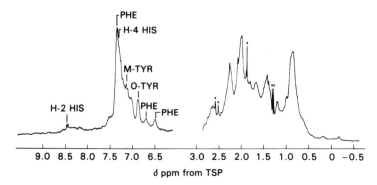

Figure 2. The 250 MHz ^{1}H-NMR Spectrum of Apo-Troponin-C; [troponin-C] *ca.* 1.0 mM, 0.2 M KCl, pH = 6.6. Resonance assignments to the H-2 protons of histidine-125, the ortho and meta protons of tyrosines-10 and -109, and two uniquely shifted phenylalanine are indicated. Resonance peaks due to impurities in the aliphatic region are labeled (X).

acid residues. That the apo-protein posesses a considerable amount of secondary structure has also been shown by CD studies [70]. Furthermore, studies on tryptic fragments of troponin-C have suggested that in the absence of calcium there are regions of α-helix which are incompletely formed [30]. The NMR and CD data are consistent with the proposal that the apo-protein is in a loosely folded conformation with regions of secondary structure which are incompletely formed. There is, however, a unique region of structure, indicated by the anomalously shifted resonances in the NMR spectrum.

C. Effect of Calcium Binding on the Conformation of Troponin-C

The calcium binding studies of Potter and Gergely [29] clearly indicate that troponin-C binds calcium at two classes of sites, two high affinity sites ($K_A = 2 \times 10^7$ M^{-1}) which competitively bind magnesium, and two lower affinity calcium specific sites ($K_A = 3 \times 10^5$ M^{-1}). Most of the early studies indicated that the calcium-induced conformational change in troponin-C occurred as a function of calcium occupancy of the high affinity sites. These studies were not able to detect further conformational changes which could be attributed to the binding of calcium at the low affinity sites. This was difficult to reconcile with the known physiological importance of calcium binding at the low affinity sites [29,71]. The sensitivity of NMR to subtle changes in the tertiary structure of proteins made it a particularly attractive technique for the observation of small structural changes which might be attributed to calcium occupancy of the low affinity sites.

A complete calcium titration of troponin-C, monitored by ^{1}H-NMR, was performed [68]. The NMR spectra of troponin-C at various stages of the titration were analyzed as a function of the fractional occupancy of specific binding sites. In this analysis the populations P_1 and P_2 correspond to the fraction of protein with one and two high affinity sites occupied, while P_3 and P_4 correspond to the fraction of protein with one and two low affinity sites occupied. A two step conformational change is demonstrated when calcium dependent spectral shifts are correlated with the actual occupancy of the high and low affinity sites. The first change is completed as the population P_1 and P_2 approach unity. A second change is manifest as populations P_3 and P_4 increase. The ability to observe apparently distinct conformational transitions due to two classes of calcium binding sites is a consequence of the large difference in the dissociation constants between the two sets of sites.

A number of spectral changes are observed as calcium is added to the protein to saturate the high affinity sites (Figure 3a-d). The principal phenylalanine resonance at 7.34 ppm decreases in intensity in parallel with an increase in intensity of the upfield phenylalanine resonance at 7.19 ppm. At the point where $P_1 \sim P_2 \sim 1$ the intensities of the two resonances are approximately equal. The change in the relative intensities indicates that a number of phenylalanine residues are entering an environment different from that of the bulk solvent. It is also observed that the high field shifted phenylalanine resonances are not affected by calcium binding at the high affinity sites. The same is true for the two high field shifted aliphatic resonances [68]. Other spectral characteristics of the first stage conformational transition have been defined by Levine et al. [72]. The histidine residue exhibits two resonances whose relative intensities reflect the fraction of protein with calcium bound at the high affinity sites. Such behavior is characteristic of a slow rate of exchange between the conformations of the calcium free and calcium bound protein. A similar behavior is also seen for one of the ortho proton resonances of a tyrosine residue. This has been attributed to a change in the environment of tyrosine-109. Additional characteristics of the first stage conformational transition include a broadening of side chain methylene resonances of acidic amino acid residues and a broadening of the α-CH proton resonances. A number of aliphatic residues are also affected by the binding of calcium at the high affinity sites as indicated by increased linewidths in the

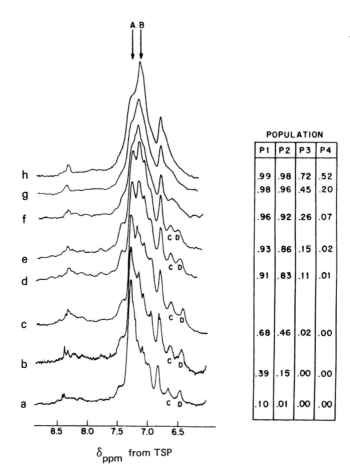

Figure 3.   Aromatic Region of the 250 MHz ^{1}H-NMR Spectrum of Troponin-C as a function of Site Population; [troponin-C] *ca.* 1.0 mM, 0.2 M KCl, pH 6.6. The fractional populations, P_i, of binding sites are given for each spectrum (see text and reference 68). The populations were calculated based on the binding parameters of Potter and Gergely [29]; for the high affinity sites, n = 2, K_A = 2.1 x 10^7 M^{-1}; and, for the low affinity sites, n = 2, K_A = 3.2 x 10^5 M^{-1}. (Adapted with permission from K. B. Seamon, D. J. Hartshorne and A. A. Bothner-By, *Biochemistry, 16*:4039 (1977); copyright American Chemical Society).

aliphatic region. The line broadening is due to an increased dispersion in chemical shifts and/or restricted rotation of the aliphatic side chains.

The first conformational transition (which corresponds to the addition of two mole equivalents of calcium to troponin-C) is due almost entirely to the binding of calcium at the high affinity sites. The thermal stability of the protein is increased after loading of the high affinity sites and appears to be almost identical to that of the protein with all four sites occupied [72]. These results, with respect to the first stage conformational transition, indicate that troponin-C $(Ca^{2+})_2$ has a more structured conformation than that of the apo-protein. This is a result of an increased α-helical content in conjunction with increased interactions between various regions of the polypeptide chain resulting in a more stable structure.

The spectral changes which are observed to occur as the low affinity sites become occupied (Figure 3d-h) suggest that a second calcium-induced conformational change takes place. The second transition is characterized by a continued increase in phenylalanine resonance intensity appearing upfield. The shift upfield appears to be similar to that which is seen during the first stage conformational transition and is interpreted as being due to increased sampling of a hydrophobic environment by the phenylalanine rings. An increase in helical content of the protein has also been ascribed to calcium occupancy of the low affinity sites, although its magnitude is less than that due to binding at the high affinity sites [73]. Even though the overall conformational change resulting from occupancy of the low affinity sites is not as dramatic as that attributed to the high affinity sites, the continued shift of the principal phenylalanine resonance suggests that the protein is indeed experiencing a further "tightening" of its structure.

One striking spectral characteristic of the second conformational transition is the downfield shift of the phenylalanine resonances (labelled C and D in Figure 3) which appear outside of the main phenylalanine peak. A linear relationship between the downfield shift of resonance D and P_3 exists which indicates that occupancy of the low affinity sites is responsible for this spectral change. A similar downfield shift is observed for two upfield shifted aliphatic residues [68]. These uniquely shifted resonances are observed in the spectrum of the apo-protein and are characteristic of a region of close hydrophobic interactions in the protein structure. Thus, in contrast to the behavior of the principal phenylalanine resonance, the upfield shifted aromatic and aliphatic resonances suggest a loss of a region of tertiary structure upon occupation of the low affinity sites. The NMR results clearly demonstrate that calcium binding at the physiologically important low affinity sites does induce a significant change in the protein's solution conformation which is presumably necessary for the expression of the biological activity of troponin-C.

D.   Effect of Magnesium on the Conformation of Troponin-C

Magnesium is able to bind competitively at the high affinity sites of
troponin-C [29]. Conformational changes, which are qualitatively similar
to those of calcium binding but of lesser magnitude, have been associated
with this binding. Since the intracellular magnesium concentration (2-3
mM) is high enough to saturate the high affinity sites ($K_d \sim 2.5 \times 10^{-4}$ M)
it is important to determine the effect of magnesium binding on the
solution conformation of troponin-C.

Magnesium binding to troponin-C results in NMR spectral changes
qualitatively similar to those associated with calcium binding at the high
affinity sites [68]. This is characterized by almost equal intensities of the
two main phenylalanine peaks. The downfield shifts of the upfield shifted
phenylalanine and aliphatic resonances, which are associated with calcium
binding at the low affinity sites, do not occur at high magnesium ion
concentrations thus confirming the calcium specificity of the low affinity
sites. As discussed by Levine et al. [74], the two conformers of troponin-C
with calcium and magnesium at the high affinity sites although qualitatively similar are not identical and do display distinct differences. A small
magnesium-induced shift in one of the upfield shifted phenylalanine resonances is observed. However, it is not as large as that induced by calcium
binding at the low affinity sites. The lack of effect of magnesium on the
high field phenylalanine and aliphatic resonances indicate that the region
of tertiary structure associated with the low affinity sites is not significantly
altered by magnesium binding.

These results further support the physiological importance of the low
affinity binding sites. In the resting muscle cell troponin-C should be
predominantly in the conformation with the high affinity sites occupied by
magnesium. The significant conformational difference upon excitation of
the cell and subsequent increase in free calcium is probably that associated
with the binding of calcium at the low affinity sites.

E.   Studies on Peptide Fragments of Troponin-C

Experiments with peptide fragments of troponin-C have contributed significantly to the identification of regions in the protein involved not only
in calcium binding but also involved in interactions with the other subunits. Thus, some fragments retain calcium binding activity and are able to
bind to troponin-I [30].

A cyanogen bromide fragment, CB-9, has been isolated which consists of the 52 amino acid residues between Lys-84 and Met-135 [75]. This fragment contains the S_3 binding site (Figure 1) which undergoes a calcium-induced conformational change [76]. The solution conformations of this fragment display many qualitative similarities to those of the native troponin-C. Birnbaum and Sykes [77] have studied the calcium-dependent conformations of the peptide using ^{1}H-NMR. The spectrum of the apo-CB-9 fragment is suggestive of a random coil exhibiting no spectral shifts characteristic of extensive tertiary structure. The phenylalanine and tyrosine-109 ring proton resonances appear at positions consistent with random coil conformers. There is also an absence of ring current shifted aliphatic peaks. Upon binding calcium spectral changes, such as the appearance of ring current shifted aliphatic resonances, and an upfield shift of some of the phenylalanine resonances are observed to occur which are suggestive of hydrophobic interactions between phenylalanine and aliphatic residues. Tyrosine-109 is also affected by the transition with the ortho and meta proton resonances shifting upfield and reversing their relative resonance positions. These observations are in agreement with studies by Nagy et al. [76], in which it was determined that the binding of calcium results in the formation of a helical segment involving residues 94-102. It is also noted that the upfield shifted phenylalanine and aliphatic resonances that are observed in the spectrum of apo-troponin-C, and are sensitive to the binding of calcium at the low affinity sites, are not observed in the spectrum of the apo-CB-9 fragment.

It has been demonstrated that peptide fragments produced by proteolysis of troponin-C with thrombin or trypsin retain the ability to bind calcium [30]. In the presence of calcium, trypsin cleaves troponin-C at lysine-84 and lysine-9 effectively splitting the protein into two large fragments each of which contains two calcium binding sites. Cleavage by thrombin results in two fragments one of which contains three binding sites, S_1-S_3, and which retains the ability to bind calcium. A ^{1}H-NMR comparison of the tryptic peptide TR1 which contains the two low affinity sites, the thrombin peptide, and native troponin-C has been made by Evans et al. [78]. The results indicate that in the absence of calcium all three polypeptides contain similar regions of structure characterized by two upfield shifted phenylalanine peaks and two upfield shifted aliphatic peaks. The resonances show similar thermal behavior indicating that the close hydrophobic interactions which are responsible for these resonances do not rely on long range interactions with other regions of the protein. The binding of calcium produces a downfield shift of the resonances which has previously been identified with calcium occupancy of the low affinity sites. The downfield shift observed for the peptide fragments is larger than seen in native troponin-C. This is attributed to the absence of interactions with regions of the protein which are missing in the individual peptides. These results confirm that the uniquely shifted resonances in the apo-troponin-C are due to residues involved in close hydrophobic interactions associated with the low affinity binding sites.

The results with the peptide fragments are consistent with the results on the intact troponin-C. In the absence of calcium there is little tertiary structure except for a region of close interactions associated with the low affinity sites. The binding of metals results in a compacting and structuring of the proteins principally due to binding at the high affinity sites. The binding of calcium at the low affinity sites results in more subtle changes in the protein structure and affects the spatial orientation between the two low affinity calcium binding domains.

III. CALMODULIN

A. Function of Calmodulin as a Calcium Regulatory Protein

Calmodulin was originally isolated as a protein activator of 3', 5'-cyclic nucleotide phosphodiesterase [79]. Subsequently, a wide variety of enzyme systems have been described which are activated or modulated by interaction with a calcium-calmodulin complex. These include brain adenylate cyclase [80,81], myosin light chain kinase isolated from smooth muscle [82] and brain [83], phosphorylase kinase [84], Ca^{2+}, Mg^{2+}-ATPase [85-87], and a number of other diverse enzyme systems [45]. Regulation by calmodulin is not limited to mammalian systems; an NAD-dependent kinase isolated from plants which can be stimulated by cal-modulin has been described [88]. Calmodulins isolated from various vertebrate species appear to be almost identical and only a few amino acid differences have been noted in calmodulin isolated from invertebrates [45]. It is clear that calmodulin is an ubiquitous calcium-dependent regula-tory protein which acts to regulate numerous enzyme systems by render-ing them sensitive to transient changes in free calcium ion concentration.

The smooth muscle contractile event in chicken gizzard is completely dependent on the activation of the myosin light chain kinase by calcium and calmodulin [82]. In this regard calmodulin plays a role similar to that of troponin-C, that is, it acts as the intracellular calcium receptor protein and mediates the effects of a transient increase in free calcium on the contractile event. One notable difference between troponin-C and calmodulin is that skeletal actomyosin is the only enzyme system which is regulated in vivo by troponin-C while calmodulin regulates a number of different systems. The binding of calmodulin to these enzymes depends on its ability to bind calcium. It has been demonstrated that calmodulin binds to adenylate cyclase [14] and phosphodiesterase [13] only in the presence of calcium. It is the enzyme calmodulin calcium complex which represents the activated system. Therefore, as with troponin-C, it is the binding of calcium to the regulatory protein and a subsequent change in its conformation that is the initial step in the activation event.

B. Conformation of Apo-Calmodulin

The ^{1}H-NMR spectrum of apo-calmodulin (Figure 4) is not typical of a random coil spectrum indicating that the protein retains considerable structure in the absence of metal ions. The tyrosine-138 ortho and meta proton resonances are shifted upfield and exhibit almost identical chemical shifts which reflect their unique environment. The tyrosine-99 protons exhibit a resonance pattern more typical of a solvent exposed tyrosine ring. The evidence for tertiary structure in the apo-protein is a phenylalanine resonance which is shifted out of the main phenylalanine peak, the position of the tyrosine-138 resonances, and upfield shifted aliphatic resonances. The bulk of the phenylalanine resonance intensity is in two peaks, the larger of which appears at a chemical shift position characteristic of solvent exposed phenylalanine rings. The smaller peak is shifted *ca.* 0.3 ppm upfield and indicates a more structured environment for some of the aromatic rings. The aliphatic region of the spectrum displays a number of

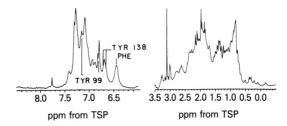

Figure 4. The 360 MHz ^{1}H-NMR Spectrum of Apo-Bovine Brain Calmodulin; [calmodulin] *ca.* 1.0 mM, 0.2 M KCl, pH 7.5. Resonance assignments to histidine-107, tyrosine-99 and 138, trimethyllysine-115, and uniquely shifted phenylalanine resonances are indicated. (Adapted with permission from K. B. Seamon, *Biochemistry, 19*:207 (1980); copyright American Chemical Society).

ring current shifted methyl resonances indicative of close interactions between aromatic rings and aliphatic side chains. The large single peak at 3.12 ppm is due to the trimethylamino group of ϵ-trimethyllysine-115. The narrow linewidth of this resonance suggests that this residue is solvent exposed and not buried in the interior of the protein.

These data are in agreement with previous work on the solution conformation of calmodulin demonstrating that apo-calmodulin has considerable secondary structure. Tyrosine-138 is in a unique environment, as indicated by its high pK of 11.3 and its sensitivity to chemical modifying agents, whereas tyrosine-99 has the properties of a solvent exposed tyrosine ring [89]. There exists a region of tertiary structure with hydrophobic interactions between aromatic rings and aliphatic side chains, as evidenced by the presence of high field shifted phenylalanine resonances and the ring current shifted methyl resonances.

C. Ca^{2+}-induced Conformations

Early physical and chemical studies on calmodulin demonstrated that the binding of calcium by the protein was accompanied by a change in its conformation [90-94]. Many of these calcium induced changes were similar to those associated with troponin-C. The assignment of conformational transitions to the occupancy of specific calcium binding sites was difficult due to conflicting values reported for calcium ion dissociation constants. Although all studies agreed that calmodulin bound four moles of calcium, the relative number of high and low affinity sites has differed [91,92,94,95]. Some studies have also suggested that monovalent cations and divalent cations such as magnesium antagonize the binding of calcium by calmodulin [92].

Calcium titrations of apo-calmodulin were carried out and the ^{1}H-NMR spectral changes were analyzed in terms of the molar ratio of calcium to calmodulin [96]. A detailed analysis of the spectral changes in terms of specific site occupancy was not carried out because of the discrepancies in binding constants which have been reported. The aromatic region of the spectrum of calmodulin at various stages of calcium binding is shown in Figure 5. The binding of calcium to calmodulin, as revealed by spectral shifts, was rationalized in terms of a sequential binding of pairs of calcium ions at two classes of sites. The first stage conformational transition due to the binding of two calcium ions was accompanied by the following spectral changes:

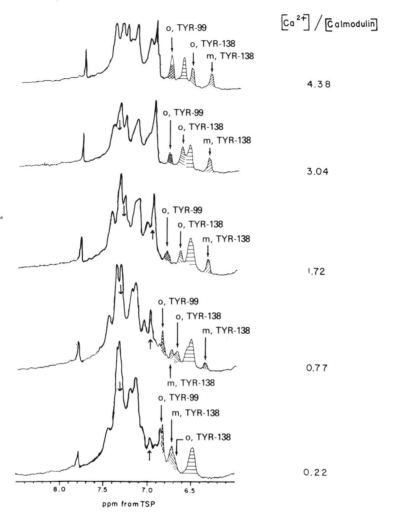

Figure 5. The 360 MHz ^{1}H-NMR Spectra of Bovine Brain Calmodulin as a Function of Calcium Content; [calmodulin] *ca.* 1.0 mM, 0.2 M KCl, pH 7.5. Calcium was added sequentially to a sample of apo-calmodulin as described [96]. The calcium to calmodulin molar ratio is indicated to the right of the spectra. The resonances assigned to the ortho protons of tyrosines-99 and 138 and the meta protons of tyrosine-138 are labeled. The slow exchange behavior of the meta protons of tyrosine-138 is clearly shown in the spectrum with $[Ca^{2+}]/[calmodulin] = 0.77$, where the two tyrosine-138 meta proton resonances originating from the two conformers are separately labeled. Arrows in the main phenylalanine peak indicate intensity changes. (Adapted with permission from K. B. Seamon, *Biochemistry, 19*:207 (1980); copyright American Chemical Society).

1. The tyrosine-138 meta proton resonance appears upfield increasing in intensity in parallel with a decrease in its intensity at its position in the spectrum of the apo-protein. This change is fully manifest at a calcium to calmodulin molar ratio of *ca*. 2 and the resonance is not affected by further additions of calcium.

2. The tyrosine-138 ortho proton resonance shifts upfield *ca*. 20 Hz.

3. The high field shifted phenylalanine resonance shifts downfield to 6.55 ppm.

4. The tyrosine-99 ortho proton resonance shifts upfield 20 Hz and is not affected by calcium in excess of a molar ratio of 2.32.

5. There is a redistribution of intensity in the main peak of phenylalanine intensity with more resonance intensity appearing upfield.

6. The ϵ-trimethyllysine resonance appears upfield 6.5 Hz in parallel with the decrease in intensity of the peak at the resonance position of the apo-protein. This change is also fully manifest at a molar ratio of calcium to calmodulin of $\sim$ 2.

These spectral changes indicate that a large change in the environment of a number of amino acid residues is taking place due to the binding of two moles of calcium by calmodulin. This is consistent with other studies on calmodulin which report that the large change in conformation due to calcium binding was almost complete at a molar ratio of calcium to calmodulin of $\sim$ 2 [97]. Since the tyrosine-138 meta proton resonance and the ϵ-trimethyllysine resonance are not affected by the addition of a third and fourth calcium it would seem that a specific conformational transition affecting these residues is due to the binding of calcium at two nearly equivalent sites. This structural change is associated with an increase in helical content as well as a change in the environment of aromatic amino acid residues. The NMR data suggest that the structural change involves a large part of the polypeptide chain and is characterized by an increase in tertiary structure through increased interactions between nonpolar amino acid residues in the interior of the protein. This first stage conformational transition is also accompanied by a perturbation of resonances associated with a unique region of tertiary structure present in the apo-calmodulin; the upfield shifted phenylalanine resonances. This region is perturbed in such a way as to decrease the relative proximity of 1 to 2 phenylalanines and 2 to 3 aliphatic side chains which are responsible for the uniquely shifted resonances.

A second conformational transition is observed during the addition of a third and fourth calcium to calmodulin. This second transition is indicated by the following spectral changes:

1. The tyrosine-138 ortho proton resonance continues to shift upfield appearing downfield of the tyrosine-138 meta proton resonance.

2. The upfield shifted phenylalanine resonance shifts downfield with part of its intensity appearing at 6.65 ppm and part shifting further downfield and appearing at the same chemical shift as the tyrosine-99 ortho proton resonances. These results demonstrate that the upfield shifted phenylalanine resonance in the spectrum of apo-calmodulin corresponds to two sets of resonances appearing at the same chemical shift.

3. A further redistribution of intensity in the main phenylalanine peak is evident with more intensity appearing upfield.

No further spectral changes are observed when calcium is added in excess of a molar ratio of four. These spectral shifts provide evidence that a second conformational transition is occurring due to the binding of a third and fourth calcium ion. This change in conformation is not as dramatic as that associated with the binding of the first two calcium ions but it does represent a significant change in tertiary structure. The continued redistribution of phenylalanine intensity could be due to a further increase in helical content or to more interactions of the aromatic rings in a nonsolvent environment. The continued downfield shift of the unique phenylalanine resonances is due to a further change in the environment of these residues which place them in a less structured environment.

Recent studies by Crouch and Klee [97], carried out under similar conditions of ionic strength and pH as the NMR studies, indicate that calmodulin binds calcium at four sites with different affinities. The two high affinity binding sites display positive cooperativity. These results are clearly compatible with the NMR results which also suggest that calmodulin contains two classes of sites. It is also reported that the calcium dependent changes in the near CD spectrum and UV spectrum of calmodulin are essentially complete when the two high affinity sites are occupied while the activation of cyclic nucleotide phosphodiesterase requires that the third and fourth binding sites be occupied [97]. This suggests that the second conformational transition probably is the physiologically important structural change in calmodulin necessary for the activation of at least the cyclic nucleotide phosphodiesterase.

D. Ca^{2+}-Dependent Perturbation of Tyrosine-138

The perturbations of the tyrosine-138 resonances appear to be the result of more than one change in the local environment around the tyrosine ring.

It is evident that calcium binding to the high affinity sites of calmodulin affects both the ortho and meta resonances of tyrosine-138 although they reflect different rates for the conformational transition. The meta resonances exhibit slow exchange behavior which allows one to set an upper limit on the rate constant for the associated conformational transition from the relationship, $k \leq 2\pi\Delta\nu$ corresponds to the separation constant in s^{-1} and $\Delta\nu$ corresponds to the separation in Hz for the two resonances in slow exchange. Similarly, it is possible to place a lower limit on the rate constant derived from the fast exchange behavior of the ortho resonance from the relationship $k \geq 2\pi\Delta\nu$ where $\Delta\nu$ corresponds to the separation in Hz between the initial and final resonance positions. Estimated rate constants which can be associated with the first conformational transition were calculated based on the above considerations. These are given in Table I.

If it is assumed that binding of calcium to the high affinity sites is diffusion controlled ($k_{on} \sim 10^8 M^{-1}s^{-1}$) and that the kinetic constants in Table I are related to the first order rate constant (k_{off}) for the decomposition of the calcium-calmodulin complex then the thermodynamic association constants for the formation of the complex can be estimated. Based on the kinetic constants obtained from the behavior of the tyrosine-138 resonances association constants for the high affinity sites are estimated to be between 1.2×10^5 M^{-1} and 8.8×10^5 M^{-1}. This result is in excellent agreement with the association constants of 3×10^5 M^{-1} and 8.6×10^5 M^{-1} determined by Crouch and Klee [97]. However, the kinetic constant associated with the trimethyllysine resonance leads to an over estimation (2.5×10^6 M^{-1}) of the association constant for the high affinity sites. This fact may indicate that the off rate for calcium from the site(s) ultimately affecting the resonances is faster than the actual conformational transition

TABLE I

**Estimated Kinetic Constants for the
First Stage Conformational Transition**

Estimated k (s⁻¹)	Resonance
≤ 814	tyrosine-138 (meta protons)
≥ 113	typrosine-138 (ortho protons)
≤ 40	ϵ-trimethylysine-115

or that the on rate for calcium is less than diffusion controlled. Furthermore, the rate constants determined from the ϵ-trimethyllysine resonance and the tyrosine-138 ortho resonance are contradictory and suggest that they may be reflecting different conformational transitions. Since tyrosine-138 is in the S_4 binding site the fast exchange behavior of the ortho proton resonance may be a direct measure of calcium exchange at the binding site and not the accompanying conformational transition. For instance, the neutralization of neighboring carboxyl groups or the replacement of potassium counterions with calcium may be responsible for the behavior of the ortho proton resonance. If this were true, then the binding constant determined from the behavior of the ortho protons would be a good estimate of the intrinsic binding constant. Since the behavior of resonances in slow exchange place only an upper limit on the rate constant for the environmental change, it is conceivable that the transition affecting the tyrosine-138 meta protons is governed by a much smaller rate constant than that associated with the ortho protons. The results of titrating apo-calmodulin with protons or magnesium ions seem to justify this conclusion. As magnesium is added to apo-calmodulin the ortho proton resonance exhibits an upfield shift and the meta proton resonance shifts downfield (Figure 6). The upfield shift of the ortho protons is similar to that seen during the first stage calcium induced conformational transition. The shift downfield of the meta proton resonance however in no way resembles the behavior of the resonance due to calcium binding. Similar behavior is exhibited by the resonances during the course of a proton titration (Figure 7). The meta resonance shifts downfield accompanied by a very small upfield shift of the ortho proton resonance. These results are consistent with the following conclusions concerning tyrosine-138. The anomolous upfield shift of the meta proton resonance is due at least in part to an environment determined by free carboxyl groups. Proton binding or magnesium binding to these groups affects the environment around the meta protons, resulting in a downfield shift of the resonance closer to its normal unperturbed resonance position. The slow exchange behavior and large change in chemical shift of the meta protons due to calcium binding is therefore associated with a large conformational transition which is not induced by proton or magnesium binding. The upfield shift of the ortho protons is probably more closely associated with the exchange of metals and/or protons at a binding site and the kinetics of the environmental change affecting these protons is related to the dynamics of the metal ion exchange at the binding site.

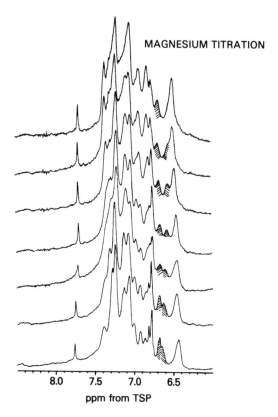

Figure 6. Magnesium Titration of Apo-Calmodulin; [calmodulin] ≅ 1.5 mM, 0.2 M KCl, pH 7.5. Magnesium was added in increments to apocalmodulin. The 360 MHz ^{1}H-NMR spectra are displayed from the bottom of the figure to the top increasing from no magnesium to *ca.* 10 mM free magnesium. The tyrosine-138 ortho (upfield,) and meta (downfield,) proton resonances are indicated. (Adapted with permission from K. B. Seamon, (*Biochemistry, 19*:207 (1980); copyright American Chemical Society).

IV. STRUCTURAL CONCLUSIONS CONCERNING TROPONIN-C AND CALMODULIN

A number of features of the ^{1}H-NMR studies allow a close examination of the predicted metal binding domains in the sequences of troponin-C and

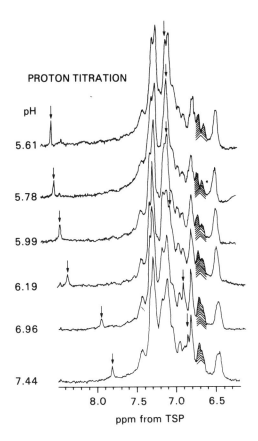

Figure 7. Proton Titration of Apo-Calmodulin; [calmodulin] ≅ 1.5 mM, 0.2 M KCl, pH 7.5. A sample of apo-calmodulin was titrated with a solution of DCl. The 360 MHz ^{1}H-NMR spectra are shown with corresponding pH values (uncorrected for deuterium isotope effects). The tyrosine-138 ortho (upfield, ⬭) and meta (downfield, ⬭) proton resonances are indicated. The histidine-107 H-2 (downfield) and H-4 (upfield) resonances are labeled by the arrows in each spectrum.

calmodulin. The NMR data can be used to define structural similarities and differences between the two proteins in solution and to determine if these structural features result in similar metal ion induced conformational transitions.

A. Locations of Calcium Binding Sites

1.   Troponin-C

The four binding domains of troponin-C have been assigned by studies on proteolytic fragments [30] and by chemical modification of carboxyl groups [31]. There is good agreement that the S_1 and S_2 sites correspond to the low affinity calcium specific binding sites and the S_3 and S_4 sites are the high affinity calcium, magnesium binding sites. Unambiguous assignments of resonances in the spectra of troponin-C have been made only for histidine-125 and the two tyrosines, 10 and 109. Histidine-125 is in a five residue sequence that connects the S_3 and S_4 sites. The pK of the histidine decreases from 7.2 to 6.6 in going from apo-troponin-C to calcium saturated troponin-C. Furthermore, it has been demonstrated that the histidine ring proton resonances are affected by calcium binding principally at the high affinity sites [72]. These data are consistent with the placement of histidine-125 in a region of the protein which is associated with the high affinity sites.

Tyrosines-10 and 109 exhibit resonance positions characteristic of solvent exposed tyrosine rings. This is in agreement with chemical modification studies which indicate that the tyrosine rings are predominantly in an aqueous solvent environment [69]. Tyrosine-109 is placed in the S_3 binding site and is predicted to participate in calcium coordination. The homologous position in carp-parvalbumin is occupied by phenylalanine-57 which participates in calcium binding through its peptide carbonyl with its aromatic ring directed toward the solvent. If tyrosine-109 of troponin-C occupies a similar position as phenylalanine-57 of carp-parvalbumin then it is predicted that the tyrosine ring would also be directed toward the solvent. Assuming a relatively unrestricted environment for tyrosine-109 in apo-troponin-C it would also be predicted that calcium binding at the S_3 site would have only a small overall effect on the tyrosine ring. In fact a slight broadening of the tyrosine-109 resonance due to calcium binding at the high affinity sites has been detected by Levine et al. [72] and has been attributed to decreased mobility of the tyrosine ring. A similar effect of magnesium has also been noted [74] and this would be expected as the S_3 site in one of the high affinity sites which competitively binds magnesium.

Further evidence that the S_3 binding site is a high affinity site is found in studies on troponin-C in which cysteine-98 has been derivatized with a S-trifluoroacetonyl group [68]. Cysteine-98 resides in the helical region immediately preceding the S_3 binding loop. As a consequence of its position near the S_3 site it would be predicted that cysteine-98 would be affected similarly by both calcium and magnesium. The ^{19}F NMR spectrum of apo-S-trifluoroacetonyl-troponin-C exhibits a single resonance that is shifted downfield identically upon addition of either saturating amounts of calcium or magnesium. These data support the assignment of the S_3 binding domain as a calcium, magnesium binding site and further suggest that this region of structure is not substantially altered by calcium binding at the low affinity sites.

Since specific resonance assignments for amino acid residues in the S_1 and S_2 binding domains have not been made, it is difficult to confirm the identification of the S_1 and S_2 sites as calcium-specific low affinity sites by proton NMR. A comparison of the spectral characteristics of native troponin-C with those of the peptide fragments which contain only sites S_1 and S_2 however provide evidence that these sites are indeed the low affinity binding sites [78]. This is possible because of the presence of unique high field shifted phenylalanine and aliphatic resonances that appear at identical chemical shifts in the spectra of native troponin-C and the peptides which contain the S_1 and S_2 sites. These resonances have been associated with structural rearrangements which occur as the low affinity sites become occupied. The two aliphatic residues have been assigned to a leucine and an isoleucine residue [78]. There are five phenylalanines, four isoleucines, and four leucine residues in the tryptic fragment containing the S_1 and S_2 binding sites and an unambiguous assignment of the shifted resonances is presently not possible. It has been suggested that close interactions between phenylalanine residues in the A_1 and B_2 helices are responsible for the high field shifted aromatic resonances [78]. This is also indicated by the sequence homology with carp-parvalbumin which predicts that phe-19, phe-76 and phe-23 phe-72 will be in close contact in the interior of troponin-C.

2. Calmodulin

The NMR data clearly indicate a sequential binding of calcium at binding sites resulting in at least two distinct conformational transitions; the first due to the binding of two calcium ions. In order to rationalize the two step conformational transition in terms of four independent and equal binding sites (as has been reported [94]) a situation must be envisioned where the calcium occupancy of any two of the four sites results in an identical conformation at a unique region of structure of calmodulin that is not further affected by the occupancy of more than two sites. Although the NMR results, as well as any physical measurements, cannot distinguish between the situation described above and that of sequential binding at different classes of sites, as is the case for troponin-C, the equivalency of all four sites with respect to the binding of the first two calcium ions seems unlikely. Therefore, it is argued that the NMR results and the binding data of Crouch and Klee [97] are most consistent with a sequential binding of calcium at different classes of binding sites.

There is no chemical data which allows an assignment of the high and low affinity sites of calmodulin. However, it is possible to distinguish NMR spectral characteristics associated with the binding of calcium at high and low affinity sites. It is also fortunate that some of the spectral shifts observed with calcium binding at the high affinity sites are associated with assigned resonances. This allows a tentative identification of the high affinity sites and, by implication, the low affinity sites.

Tyrosine-99 occurs in the S_3 binding loop of calmodulin where it is predicted to participate in calcium coordination through its peptide carbonyl moiety. It occupies a position homologous to tyrosine-109 of troponin-C and displays similar calcium induced spectral behavior, a slight upfield shift which is essentially complete at a molar ratio of calcium to protein of *ca.* 2. As exemplified by tyrosine-109 of troponin-C, this behavior implies that tyrosine-99 is located at the binding site. These data and other published work [89] suggest that the tyrosine-99 ring is experiencing a relatively solvent accessible environment which is not dramatically altered by the occupancy of the S_3 site by calcium. Since the spectral shift of the tyrosine-99 ortho proton resonance is fully manifest at a calcium to calmodulin molar ratio of *ca.* 2, it is predicted that the S_3 binding site is one of the two high affinity binding sites.

The spectral behavior of the trimethylamino resonance of ϵ-trimethyllysine-115 also supports the assignment of the S_3 site as a high affinity binding site and further suggests that the S_4 binding site is a high affinity binding site. The resonance reflects a conformational change occuring as a result of calcium binding at the first two sites suggesting that ϵ-trimethyllysine-115 is near the two high affinity sites. ϵ-Trimethyllysine-115 is placed in a link region connecting the B_3 and A_4 helices of the S_3 and S_4 binding domains, respectively. If the S_3 and S_4 sites were high affinity binding sites then the ϵ-trimethyllysine-115 should be affected principally by the binding of calcium at these two sites. This is substantiated by the NMR data. It is also interesting to note that ϵ-trimethyllysine-115 is placed at a position similar to that of histidine-125 in troponin-C which has been reported to reflect the binding of calcium at the high affinity sites of troponin-C.

Although tyrosine-138 is in the S_4 binding site, it is not predicted to participate in calcium coordination. The sequence homology predicts that tyrosine-138 interacts with other nonpolar amino acid residues in the interior of the protein. This unique environment for tyrosine-138 is certainly consistent with the chemical shifts of the ring. It has been demonstrated that the meta proton resonance of tyrosine-138 reflects the large conformational transition which accompanies the binding of calcium at the high affinity sites. This is consistent with the S_4 site being a high affinity calcium binding site. The ortho proton resonance, however, is sensitive to calcium binding at high and low affinity sites. If the tyrosine ring is buried in the interior of the protein due to the first conformational transition then the spectral shift of the ortho proton resonance observed during the low affinity site conformational transition may represent subtle alterations in the hydrophobic interior of the protein. The identification of the S_4 site as a high affinity calcium binding site is based principally on the proximity of tyrosine-138 to the site and the sensitivity of its meta proton resonances to calcium binding. The possibility that the meta proton resonances are affected by occupancy of, for instance, the S_3 binding site cannot be ruled out. This would require that structural information be transmitted between sites.

There are no easily assignable resonances that are identified with the low affinity site conformational change. This change is characterized by spectral shifts observed for the high field shifted phenylalanine resonances, the tyrosine-138 ortho proton resonance, and changes in the main peak of phenylalanine intensity. By analogy with troponin-C it is also predicted that the upfield shifted phenylalanine resonances of calmodulin might originate from interactions between phe-16 and phe-65 or phe-12 and phe-68 in the A_1 and B_2 helices associated with the two sites, S_1 and S_2, respectively.

B. Structural Comparison Between Troponin-C and Calmodulin

1. Conformation of the Metal-Free Proteins

Both troponin-C and calmodulin retain considerable structure in the absence of metals. These structures are presumably extended conformations with incompletely formed helical regions. Both proteins contain a localized region of tertiary structure which, at least in troponin-C, can be directly associated with the low affinity sites. This region in troponin-C is characterized by NMR resonances originating from approximately two phenylalanines and two aliphatic residues. In contrast, the same region in calmodulin is indicated by resonances corresponding to probably two phenylalanines and six aliphatic residues. It should be pointed out that these six aliphatic residues which appear to be in structured environments could be located in different parts of the protein's structure and may not all originate from the same local region.

Little information can be obtained concerning the structure of the binding sites in the absence of metals. However, the unique environment of tyrosine-138 in the S_4 binding site of calmodulin indicates that these regions of the polypeptide chain are not random coils. The anomolous chemical shifts displayed by the tyrosine-138 ring protons can, at least in part, be explained by the close proximity of the residue with carboxyl groups at the binding site.

2. Metal Ion Induced Conformations

The binding of calcium produces large changes in secondary and tertiary structure. These changes can be rationalized in terms of the binding of calcium at two classes of binding sites which differ in their affinities for the metal. The conformational changes which accompany calcium binding to troponin-C appear to reflect structural rearrangements that are restricted to regions of structure near the binding sites. Thus specific spectral correlates that are uniquely associated with the occupancy of both the high affinity and low affinity sites are observable. Calmodulin exhibits spectral characteristics suggestive of a more complex interplay between the low affinity sites and the high affinity sites. The high affinity site conformational transition displays two types of spectral characteristics: those that are uniquely affected by the binding of calcium at the high affinity sites and those that are affected by the binding of calcium at both the high and the low affinity sites. The residues which are responsible for the spectral characteristics affected by both binding sites are therefore in a part of the protein structure which is apparently sensitive to calcium binding at all four sites.

By analogy with troponin-C it can be predicted that certain phenylalanine interactions associated with the S_1 and S_2 binding sites of calmodulin may lead to the high field shifted phenylalanine resonances. These are affected by both the high and low affinity site conformational transitions and this suggests that structure near the S_1 and S_2 binding domains is affected by the binding of calcium at the S_3 and S_4 binding sites. Similarly, it is noted that tyrosine-138 at the S_4 binding site responds to calcium binding at all four binding sites. These results and those of Crouch and Klee [97] concerning the positive cooperativity displayed by the high affinity binding sites clearly indicate that metal binding by calmodulin is governed by more complex interactions between binding sites than that associated with troponin-C.

The structural characteristics of the conformations of the proteins with the high affinity sites occupied appear to be similar. Metal ion induced structural changes result in a more stable configuration of the protein which, at least for troponin-C and probably for calmodulin, is close to that of the fully calcium saturated protein. For both troponin-C and calmodulin the estimated rate constants for the conformational change resulting from calcium binding at the high affinity sites are slow, < 20 s^{-1} for troponin-C [72] and < 40 s^{-1} for calmodulin [96]. These rate constants are associated with the considerable rearrangement of the polypeptide chain in response to the calcium binding and therefore the transitions are believed to be too slow to be involved in the physiological regulatory events with which these proteins are involved.

The second conformational transition associated with calcium binding at the low affinity sites represents a smaller overall change in the proteins' structure than that associated with the binding at the high affinity sites. There does not seem to be as large a change in secondary structure as that associated with the occupancy of the high affinity sites. The striking characteristic of the second conformational change is the rearrangement of nonpolar amino acid residues which form a region of tertiary structure in the apo-proteins. This change is also transmitted·to structural regions of calmodulin which are more directly linked to the high affinity sites. Although this may also pertain for troponin-C, it has not been observed by NMR. The conformational transition associated with occupation of the low affinity sites is believed to be a physiologically important structural change in both proteins. This conclusion is based on both the calcium ion dependence of the observed activations of enzymes by these proteins [29,97] and the kinetics of the conformational transition. The rate constant for the low affinity site conformational transition of troponin-C is estimated to be between 230 s^{-1} and 347 s^{-1} [72] while the rate for calmodulin is > 265 s^{-1}. These correspond to rates which are fast enough to initiate physiological responses.

V. CONCLUSIONS

It is evident that the ability of ^{1}H-NMR to monitor the environment of individual atoms in a complex protein structure has permitted a more thorough assessment of the molecular details of metal ion-induced structural changes in calcium binding proteins. In particular, it is important to point out that magnetic resonance techniques not only provide information concerning individual thermodynamic states of a molecular structure but also information on the dynamics of transitions between various molecular conformations. The results reviewed here for troponin-C and calmodulin show that, while these two functionally different calcium binding proteins exhibit several striking structural similarities, there are subtle but significant differences which are detected by ^{1}H-NMR. It is anticipated that by a combination of techniques, e.g., x-ray crystallography, NMR, etc., the qualitative similarities among calcium binding proteins as well as the unique differences which define their respective physiological functions will be further elucidated.

Acknowledgments

The author's work reported for troponin-C was carried out in the laboratory of Dr. Aksel Bothner-By in collaboration with Dr. David Hartshorne. The 250 MHz NMR spectra were taken on the MPC-250 spectrometer at the Mellon Institute NMR Facility for Biomedical Studies and were supported by NIH grants RR00292, AM16532, and HL09544. The 360 MHz NMR spectra were taken at the Purdue Biomedical Magnetic Resonance Laboratory and were supported by NIH grants RR01077 and U.S. Public Health Service Research Fellowship NS-05832-01 to the author. This chapter was written while the author was a fellow in the Pharmacology Research Associate Program, sponsored by NIGMS, in the laboratory of Dr. John Daly. The author would like to thank Dr. Paul Leavis and Dr. Claude Klee for communicating results prior to publication. The advice, many discussions, and excellent editorial assistance of Dr. Richard Armstrong concerning this manuscript is gratefully acknowledged.

References

1. W. W. Douglas, *Brit. J. Pharmacol., 34*:451 (1968).
2. T. D. Pollard and R. R. Weihing, *CRC Crit. Rev. Biochem., 2*:1 (1974).
3. I. Ebashi and M. Endo, *Prog. Biophys. Mol. Biol., 18*:123 (1968).
4. J.-P. Perchellet and R. K. Sharma, *Science, 203*:1259 (1979).
5. H. Rasmussen and D. B. P. Goodman, *Physiol. Rev., 57*:421 (1977).

6. P. F. Baker, *Progr. Biophys. Mol. Biol., 24*:177 (1972).
7. H. Rasmussen, D. B. P. Goodman, and A. Tenenhouse, *CRC Crit. Rev. Biochem., 1*:95 (1972).
8. B. Katz and R. Miledi, *J. Physiol., London, 192*:407 (1967).
9. K. Von Hungen and S. Roberts, *Nature (New Biol.), 242*:58 (1973).
10. R. H. Kretsinger, *Ann. Rev. Biochem., 45*:239 (1976).
11. W. D. McCubbin, R. S. Mani, and C. M. Kay, *Biochemistry, 13*:2689 (1974).
12. R. S. Mani, W. D. McCubbin, and C. M. Kay, *Biochemistry, 13*:5003 (1974).
13. Y. Teshima and S. Kakiuchi, *Biochem. Biophys. Res. Commun., 56*:489 (1974).
14. T. J. Lynch, E. A. Tallant, and W. Y. Cheung, *Biochem. Biophys. Res. Commun., 68*:616 (1976).
15. P. Calissano, S. Alema, and P. Fasella, *Biochemistry, 13*:4553 (1974).
16. Y. Teshima and S. Kakiuchi, *J. Cyclic Nucleotide Res., 4*:219 (1978).
17. R. H. Kretsinger and C. E. Nockolds, *J. Biol. Chem., 248*:3313 (1973).
18. R. H. Kretsinger, *Int. Rev. Cytol., 46*:323 (1976).
19. P. C. Moews and R. H. Kretsinger, *J. Mol. Biol., 91*:201 (1975).
20. A. Weeds and A. McLachlan, *Nature (London), 252*:246 (1974).
21. R. H. Kretsinger in *Calcium Transport in Contraction and Secretion* (E. Carofoli, ed.), North Holland Publishing Co., New York, 1975.
22. R. H. Tufty and R. H. Kretsinger, *Science, 187*: 167 (1975).
23. J. Demaille, E. Potruge, J.-P. Capony, and J.-F. Pechere in *Calcium Binding Proteins* (W. Drabikowski, H. Strezclecka-Golaszewska, and E. Carafoli, eds.), Elsevier Publishing Co., Amsterdam, 1974, p. 643.
24. J. Parello, A. Cave, P. Puigdomenech, C. Maury, J.-P. Capony, and J.-F. Pechere, *Biochimie, 56*:61 (1974).
25. D. J. Nelson, S. J. Opella, and O. Jardetzky, *Biochemistry, 15*:5551 (1976).
26. A. Cave, C. M. Dobson, J. Parello, and R. J. P. Williams, *FEBS Lett., 65*:190 (1976).
27. W. J. Birdsall, B. A. Levine, R. J. P. Williams, J. G. Demaille, J. Haiech, and J.-F. Pechere, *Biochimie, 61*:741 (1979).
28. J. H. Collins, J. D. Potter, M. J. Horn, G. Wilshire, and N. Jackman, *FEBS Lett., 36*:268 (1973).
29. J. D. Potter and J. Gergely, *J. Biol. Chem., 250*:4628 (1975).
30. P. C. Leavis, S. S. Rosenfeld, J. Gergeley, Z. Grabarek, and W. Drabikowski, *J. Biol. Chem., 253*:5452 (1978).
31. I. L. Sin, R. Fernandes, and D. Mercola, *Biochem. Biophys. Res. Comm., 82*:1132 (1978).
32. P. C. Leavis, W. Drabikowski, S. Rosenfeld, Z. Grabarek, and J. Gergely in *Calcium Binding Proteins and Calcium Function* (R. H. Wasserman et al., eds.), Elsevier, New York, 1977, p. 281.
33. A. C. Murray and C. M. Kay, *Biochemistry, 11*:2622 (1972).
34. J.-P. Van Eerd and Y. Kawasaki, *Biochem. Biophys. Res. Commun., 47*: 859 (1972).
35. J. D. Potter, J. C. Seidel, P. C. Leavis, S. S. Lehrer, and J. Gergeley, *J. Biol. Chem., 251*:7551 (1976).

36. J. Head and S. V. Perry, *Biochem. J., 137*:145 (1974).
37. J. R. Dedman, R. L. Jackson, W. E. Schreiber, and A. R. Means, *J. Biol. Chem., 253*:343 (1978).
38. R. J. A. Grand and S. V. Perry, *FEBS Lett., 92*:137 (1978).
39. D. M. Watterson, F. Sharief, and T. C. Vanaman, *J. Biol. Chem., 255*:462 (1980).
40. T. C. Vanaman, F. Sharief, and D. M. Watterson in *Calcium Binding Proteins and Calcium Function* (R. H. Wasserman et al., eds.), Elsevier, New York, 1977, p. 167.
41. F. C. Stevens, M. Walsh, H. C. Ho, T. S. Teo, and J. H. Wang, *J. Biol. Chem., 251*:4495 (1976).
42. D. M. Watterson, W. G. Harrelson Jr., P. M. Keller, F. Sharief, and T. C. Vanaman, *J. Biol. Chem., 251*:4501 (1976).
43. M. Walsh, F. C. Stevens, J. Kuznicki, and W. Drabikowski, *J. Biol. Chem., 252*:7440 (1977).
44. W. Drabikowski, Z. Grabarek, and B. Barylko, *Biochem. Biophys. Acta, 496*:216 (1977).
45. C. B. Klee, T. H. Crouch, and P. G. Richman, *Ann. Rev. Biochem., 49*:489 (1980).
46. J. D. Potter, J. D. Johnson, J. R. Dedman, W. E. Schreiber, E. Mandel, R. L. Jackson, and A. R. Means in *Calcium-Binding Proteins and Calcium Function* (R. H. Wasserman et al., eds.), Elsevier, New York, 1977.
47. L. D. Burtnick and C. M. Kay, *FEBS Lett., 75*:105 (1977).
48. P. C. Leavis and E. L. Kraft, *Arch. Biochem. Biophys., 187*:243 (1978).
49. J.-P. Van Eerd and K. Takahashi, *Biochemistry, 15*:1171 (1976).
50. L. D. Burtnick, W. D. McCubbin, and C. M. Kay, *Can. J. Biochem., 53*:15 (1975).
51. M. T. Hincke, W. D. McCubbin, and C. M. Kay, *Can. J. Biochem., 56*:384 (1978).
52. R. H. Wasserman, C. S. Fullmer, and A. H. Taylor in *Vitamin D* (D. E. M. Lawson, ed.), Academic Press, London, 1978.
53. C. S. Fullmer and R. H. Wasserman in *Calcium Binding Proteins and Calcium Function* (R. H. Wasserman et al., eds.), Elsevier, New York, 1977.
54. A. G. Szent-Gyorgi, E. M. Szent-Kiralyi, and J. Kendrick-Jones, *J. Mol. Biol., 74*:179 (1973).
55. G. Frank and A. G. Weeds, *Eur. J. Biochem., 44*:317 (1974).
56. K. Morimoto and W. F. Harrington, *J. Mol. Biol., 88*:693 (1974).
57. R. H. Kretsinger, *CRC Crit. Rev. Biochem.*, in press (1980).
58. A. Mrakovcic, S. Oda, and E. Reisler, *Biochemistry, 18*:5960 (1979).
59. M. N. Alexis and W. B. Gratzer, *Biochemistry, 17*:2319 (1978).
60. B. W. Moore, *Scand. J. Immun.*, in press (1980).
61. T. Isobe and T. Okuyama, *Eur. J. of Biochem., 89*:379 (1978).
62. K. B. Seamon and B. W. Moore, *Trans. Amer. Soc. Neurochem.*, (1979).
63. P. Calissano, S. Alema, and P. Fasella, *Biochemistry, 13*:4553 (1974).
64. P. Calissano, B. W. Moore, and A. Friesen, *Biochemistry, 8*:4318 (1969).

65. B. W. Moore, *Int. Rev. Neurobiol., 15*:215 (1972).
66. R. Donato, F. Michetti, and N. Miani, *Brain Res., 98*:561 (1975).
67. D. A. D. Parry and J. M. Squire, *J. Mol. Biol., 75*:33 (1973).
68. K. B. Seamon, D. J. Hartshorne, and A. A. Bothner-By, *Biochemistry, 16*:4039 (1977).
69. W. D. McCubbin and C. M. Kay, *FEBS Lett., 55*:183 (1975).
70. C. C. Wu and J. T. Yang, *Biochemistry, 15*:3007 (1976).
71. A. Weber and J. M. Murray, *Physiol. Rev., 53*:612 (1973).
72. B. A. Levine, D. Mercola, D. Coffman, and J. M. Thronton, *J. Mol. Biol., 115*:743 (1977).
73. M. T. Hincke, W. D. McCubbin, and C. M. Kay, *Can. J. Biochem., 56*:384 (1978).
74. B. A. Levine, J. M. Thornton, R. Fernandes, C. M. Kelly, and D. Mercola, *Biochim. Biophys. Acta, 535*:11 (1978).
75. J. H. Collins, M. L. Greaser, J. D. Potter, and M. J. Horn, *J. Biol. Chem., 252*:6356 (1977).
76. B. Nagy, J. D. Potter, and J. Gergely, *J. Biol. Chem., 253*:5971 (1978).
77. E. R. Birnbaum and B. D. Sykes, *Biochemistry, 17*:4965 (1978).
78. J. S. Evans, B. A. Levine, P. C. Leavis, J. Gergeley, Z. Grabarek, and W. Drabikowski, *Biochim. Biophys. Acta,* in press (1980).
79. W. Y. Cheung, *Biochem. Biophys. Res. Commun., 38*:533 (1970).
80. C. O. Brostrom, Y. C. Huang, B. M. McL. Breckenridge, and D. J. Wolff, *Proc. Nat. Acad. Sci. USA, 72*:64 (1975).
81. W. Y. Cheung, L. S. Bradham, T. J. Lynch, Y. M. Lin, and E. A. Tallant, *Biochem. Biophys. Res. Commun., 66*:1055 (1975).
82. R. Dabrowska, J. M. Sherry, D. K. Aromatorio, and D. J. Hartshorne, *Biochemistry, 17*:253 (1978).
83. R. Dabrowska and D. J. Hartshorne, *Biochem. Biophys. Res. Commun., 85*:1352 (1979).
84. P. Cohen, A. Burchell, J. G. Foulkes, P. T. W. Cohen, T. C. Vanaman, and A. C. Nairn, *FEBS Lett., 92*:287 (1978).
85. H. W. Jarrett and J. Kyte, *J. Biol. Chem., 254*:8237 (1979).
86. R. M. Gopinath and F. F. Vincenzi, *Biochem. Biophys. Res. Commun., 77*:1203 (1977).
87. H. W. Jarrett and J. T. Penniston, *J. Biol. Chem., 253*:4676 (1978).
88. J. M. Anderson and M. J. Cormier, *Biochem. Biophys. Res. Commun., 84*:595 (1978).
89. P. G. Richman and C. B. Klee, *Biochemistry, 17*:928 (1978).
90. Y. P. Liu and W. Y. Cheung, *J. Biol. Chem., 251*:4193 (1976).
91. C. B. Klee, *Biochemistry, 16*:1017 (1977).
92. D. J. Wolff, P. G. Poirier, C. O. Brostrom, and M. A. Brostrom, *J. Biol. Chem., 252*:4108 (1977).
93. M. Walsh and F. C. Stevens, *Biochemistry, 17*:3924 (1978).
94. J. R. Dedman, J. D. Potter, R. L. Jackson, J. D. Johnson, and A. R. Means, *J. Biol. Chem., 252*:8415 (1977).

95. Y. M. Lin, Y. P. Liu, and W. Y. Cheung, *J. Biol. Chem., 249*:4943 (1974).
96. K. B. Seamon, *Biochemistry, 19*:207 (1980).
97. T. Crouch and C. B. Klee, *Biochemistry*, in press (1980).

INDEX